A Helpful Guide
to Reducing
Triggers for
RADS

**(Reactive Airways Dysfunction Syndrome)
and other breathing issues**
Volume 1

By Taryn Bock

Foreword by Esteemed Author Dr Katrina Malin PhD

"An Extremely Valuable and Information Guide Offering
Many Practical Solutions.." Dr Atheel Badir GP

---

*Follow my journey after I was injured at work and left with RADS
and how I used myself as a guinea pig to develop creative solutions
to survive and have a better quality of life living with RADS.*

A Helpful Guide to Reducing Triggers for

RADS

**(Reactive Airways Dysfunction Syndrome)
and other breathing issues
*Volume 1***

By Taryn Bock

Foreword by Esteemed Author Dr Katrina Malin PhD

"An Extremely Valuable and Information Guide Offering Many
Practical Solutions.." Dr Atheel Badir GP

---

*Follow my journey after I was injured at work and left with RADS
and how I used myself as a guinea pig to develop creative solutions
to survive and have a better quality of life living with RADS.*

COPYRIGHT

Copyright © 2020 by Taryn Bock

First Printing: 2020

ISBN   978-0-646-81920-4

Published by RADS Int
Melbourne, Victoria, Australia

Email: radsinternational@gmail.com

Website: www.radsinternational.com
Website: www.breathingissues.weebly.com

V41AZ

Disclaimer

Although every precaution has been taken in the preparation of this work, neither the author nor the publisher shall have any liability to any person or entity with respect to any loss or damage caused or alleged to be caused directly or indirectly by the information contained in this book.

Parts of this work are fiction and are the product of the author's imagination or are used fictitiously, and any resemblance to actual persons, living or dead, events, or locales is entirely coincidental.

In order to maintain anonymity for people the author has spoken to or had contact with, she has not used any names and may have changed places, occupations and locations as well as some identifying characteristics about their experiences.

Though every effort has been made to ensure the accuracy of information contained herein, the author Taryn Bock is not a doctor. Any information or suggestions written in this book by Taryn and or RADS Int will not be held liable for any damages, pain, suffering, loss, injury, breathing issues, health issues mental or physical whatsoever, personal injury, stress (emotional or otherwise) sickness, allegedly arising from any information, methods or suggestions in this book or any decisions that you may make as a result including without limitation, actual, incidental and/or consequential damages resulting from any claims resulting from any act or omission, including without limitation, financial loss, loss of income, death errors or omissions, or otherwise.

"A Helpful Guide to Reducing Triggers for RADS (Reactive Airways Dysfunction Syndrome) and Other Breathing Issues" is a guide and collation of suggestions only and was written to inform and not provide medical advice. The information is not to be used by you in place of any medical professional or qualified and licensed professionals' instructions or medications that work for you.

You should always consult your doctor when it comes to your personal health, and/or before you start any treatment.

What works for the author may not work for you.

Contents

Foreword

I am pleased to write a few words for Taryn who has always shown me a sense of curiosity in getting to understand what curve-ball life has thrown her way. She has always been tenacious in finding better outcomes for herself and not settling for second best.

I met Taryn in June 2013, after an incident that she had been exposed to and left her shaken to the core, the fear of something unpredictable and at that time unknown; that at any stage could compromise her ability to breathe. She would attend my office in varying emotional states and reactions, yet always open to the discussion and willing to take on responsibility to understand the science behind her psychological state and how this played a major role in her ability to cope.

Her journey to navigate her RADS, to work through the WorkCover and legal systems, while developing a plan of action for herself and with a thought of spreading her knowledge about this little understood condition. A condition that could easily be labelled psychological rather than physical. To her credit, she maintained her focus and was able to work through many obstacles as penned in her book that follows.

Her enthusiasm and sincerity to help others through sharing what she has learnt through her experiences will undoubtedly mean that others that are or about to experience RADS will be guided in a meaningful and productive way. Hopefully bypassing some of the traumas that Taryn herself has had to face.

Her story is one full of emotions, from anger to sadness and to laughter. Her compassion is genuine and her ability to encourage others, inspiring.

Dr Katrina Malin PhD
Psychologist

A word from the Author

Firstly, thank you for purchasing my book and please know that although having RADS can be life changing and extremely challenging there are always options, ideas and alternatives to help you get through this journey and you are not alone.

My book is based on my personal experience living with RADS since 2012 and while some breathing issues I experience have been life-threatening and extremely scary, I am also grateful. Grateful because life today is a lot easier to manage and I have many more good days.

This is due to changes I made, being vigilant following my new rules, implementing my strategies and working on a more positive outlook.

The aim of my book is to offer information that provides insight, suggestions and hope to others living with RADS and to shine a light on and bring awareness to RADS.

My journey living with RADS continues its roller coaster ride, delivering highs, lows and prompting me to continue creating successful solutions to reduce and/or eliminate triggers, manage my RADS and live my best life. I'm somewhat of a straight shooter, so I write from the heart and share honest experiences and snippets of my life, as well as my personal view on various subjects.

Embracing change and a new way to live was tough however, for me the rewards have been worth it, not just for reducing my triggers but overall for my quality of life.

In my mind, just because I have RADS doesn't mean I can't be productive and achieve in life. I just had to get my triggers under control, create a plan, move my goalposts a little to the left, take a bit more time out to stop and not smell the roses but the sea air and invent awesome new achievable dreams.

Have a good air day and good health to all.

Sincerely,

Taryn Bock
radsinternational@gmail.com
Founder www.radsinternational.com
www.breathingissues.weebly.com
Advocate, consultant & supporter of others living with RADS

Dedication

I would like to dedicate my book to all the brave and courageous people around the world living with RADS.

A special shout out to the hundreds of people I have personally spoken with who have RADS.

To those who were also injured at work due to *unsafe work practices* and left with RADS. Allow me to officially say something that many of us have never heard and should have been said by those responsible but most often isn't …

SO VERY SORRY YOU WERE INJURED!

INDEX

INDEX cont.

INDEX cont.

INDEX cont..

INDEX cont.

What is RADS?

From what I have read and learnt from medical professionals, RADS is the acronym for Reactive Airways Dysfunction Syndrome and is described as the onset of respiratory symptoms soon after a "one time" inhalation of a highly concentrated fume, vapor, gas or smoke which can leave the person with hypersensitivity and asthma-like symptoms.

It was difficult to come to terms with the fact that so much damage had been done from just **one breath** leaving me with injuries to my airways, vocal cords, sinuses, partial collapsed lung and scaring on my lung.

A RADS Diagnosis

I saw six doctors over seven months and each time I attended and had a breathing issue and/or was coughing, it presented *like* asthma but it would usually subside after a short time when I was in their rooms, in a clean air environment.

Although the asthma tests conducted came up negative and I had never previously had asthma, breathing issues or allergies, I was misdiagnosed each time as having asthma. I vehemently explained my breathing difficulties started *immediately* after inhaling toxic steam, laden with chemicals at work and I had *never* had breathing issues prior to that exposure. I felt I was not being heard and I became extremely frustrated, frightened and perplexed. It must have also been confusing for the doctors I saw. An early diagnosis of RADS would have saved me a lot of stress and suffering and that's why I am so passionate about education and awareness about RADS.

Looking back, I believe that due to the unique symptoms of RADS including its *unpredictability*, the fact it's not well known and that RADS can mimic asthma, I kept getting sent home with steroid inhalers for asthma that either did nothing or made my breathing worse, which was a frightening situation for me. Sadly, my breathing issues weren't subsiding and I was experiencing suffocation and felt no-one understood the level of respiratory distress I was having, it was terrifying!

So, after many months of confusion, frustration and desperation I decided I had to step up for myself and do my own due diligence. I secured a referral to a Respiratory Specialist and he did his own investigations, conducted various tests over a number of weeks and eventually diagnosed me with RADS.

Aside from the breathing issues I was experiencing, I would also feel an ongoing dull pain in my back lung and I would sound quite raspy when speaking. My stress levels were through the roof and I was suffering with anxiety and panic attacks that at times made my whole-body shake, making it difficult to even hold my phone. Some of my triggers were life-threatening and I felt overwhelmed with no-one to offload to or anyone telling me I was going to be ok and I would live through this. No words of encouragement and no medication that could help me.

The first three years were an especially difficult time, trying to understand and learn how to live with RADS. My breathing issues did not subside, I reacted each time I was exposed to strong triggers and the changing of seasons and passing of time, made no difference. I spent copious hours doing personal research on the internet trying to find any information specifically about how best to live with such reactive airways. Sadly, I found nothing. You see back then, there were no internet groups for RADS, no-one offering support and over-all, not much on the internet about this unique condition. I was alone on this journey, something many of the people I have since spoken to with RADS relate to.

Over time I realized it was up to me! I had to create my own management plan, make changes to **how** I lived, **where** I lived and changing my **mindset** all played a crucial and important role in helping me manage my RADS. Eventually, I also had the good fortune to be referred to a trusted Psychologist and she was a great support to me for my mental health.

The good news is, if I can experience such good results after doing the work, making and embracing change and having a positive mindset, then that's something to get excited about!

Let your new positive chapter begin now!

Who Can Get RADS?

Sadly, there has been an increase in people contacting me who are getting RADS from accidents at home or on private property where there has been a "one-time" exposure to a highly concentrated fume, vapor, gas or smoke. The larger majority who contact me, are those injured at work and they come from all walks of life and varying types of industry. Just everyday people going about their lives and in one breath so much can instantly change.

With all the recent fires in Australia and other fires globally, when homes, businesses, factories, cars, property and other is burnt, that can produce a multitude of harmful toxins in the smoke and potentially leave someone with RADS or some other serious respiratory issue and acute sensitivities.

Tragically, many firefighters and local residents were left with RADS after the 911 attack on the twin towers in New York, USA.

What Are Triggers?

It's my understanding triggers such as smoke, fumes, fragrant, scents, fresh ink, dust, dander, pollution etc. could cause your airways to react and give you breathing issues. There are multitudes of triggers however there are ways to reduce and remove many. When you're first diagnosed, avoiding triggers is an important and vital part of managing and successfully living with RADS and I share a lot of information about how I do that.

I am extremely sensitive and reactive to what injured me and after speaking to other people with this condition, they experience the same.

There is a comprehensive list on www.radsinternational.com under Triggers.

How Do Triggers Affect Me?

I only need one breath of a particular trigger to experience various levels of respiratory distress. Usually the first thing I notice is, I will cough like I am trying to clear my throat. When I was first injured, I was coughing for a number of weeks and it got to the point that I was worried I would crack a rib, so I made an effort to do little coughs and I would sometimes kneel on my bed with my face in my pillow coughing and fall asleep in that position out of exhaustion.

These days, I only cough when first exposed to a trigger and I believe that's my bodies automatic reaction in trying to clear it, just ongoing small coughs and at the same time my voice will go hoarse, like I have laryngitis (that's my Vocal Cord Dysfunction and what I call my bodies "warning mechanism" that I need to act) and then, depending on the exposure, my airways may start to close either slowly or very fast, making it difficult for me to breathe. This is frightening and as a result of having these unpredictable breathing issues, panic attacks, stress, high anxiety and depression became prevalent.

During my litigation I had occasions where I had to attend various doctors' appointments in the city and was exposed to strong triggers and as a result, the next day I began spitting up blood. This was extremely upsetting and distressing to me, so I asked on several occasions for my appointments to be moved out of the city or be done by via the internet but was refused. I can't put into words how shocked and angry I was because I could feel the damage it was doing being exposed to all those pollutants but if I didn't go to the appointments, it could jeopardize my case.

*(Please note, in my non-medical opinion, for the many people I have spoken to with RADS over the years where we have compared our symptoms, spitting up blood has **not** been the norm. Recently this happened again and my sinuses were extremely painful, so I was sent for tests and it showed I had acute and chronic sinusitis. This explains to me where the blood is coming from.)*

This, and sore lungs, has become "my" new normal when exposed to strong triggers or if I am in any prolonged contaminated "not good" air situation. The best way I found to heal is to stay away from the city and built-up areas, be in a clean air and non-dust environment, drink warm lemon and honey and lay in my campervan (more about my van later), preferably at the beach breathing in clean salt air, away from ALL triggers. If I couldn't get to the beach then I would lay in a clean safe room (more about safe rooms later) with an air purifier running. My recovery time could take days or weeks after a high-level exposure.

Usually after a strong exposure to a trigger my airways become extremely sensitive to items or situations I may have tolerated prior to the trigger and I have to isolate myself from everyone and everything, until my airways calm down and I begin the recovery process.

Sometimes the day after a strong trigger and difficulty breathing, I end up with what I call lung inflammation or sore lungs and it's very painful just to take a breath. It feels like I have gone 10 rounds in a boxing ring and the lining inside my lungs has been bruised. The best remedy for me is again, laying in my campervan resting at the beach and breathing in clean salt air and it's very important I lay down, as I have noticed that sitting slows down my recovery time.

If I couldn't get to the beach then I would lay in a clean safe room near my air purifier. Prior to being near the beach, I would clean out my car and drive to the forest and lay in the back of my car breathing in clean air. If I am sleeping in a room where the air is compromised, I notice I wake up with my lips pursed shut, I'm breathing through my nose and I have sore lungs and tender airways.

Another after-effect of some triggers is, that I can smell and taste that trigger down my throat and, in my saliva, the following day and/or I may have a thin film of mucus. So, my morning ritual is to always gargle and spit, sometimes with salt water or with clean water.

There were times I would sometimes feel a dull ache and lung pain in my back after exposure to particular triggers. This would disappear after a few days whenever I was at the ocean breathing in clean salt air or in a clean air environment. I also noticed that aside from serious breathing issues, certain triggers like sulphur and diesel exhaust can also cause what felt like my upper stomach to puff up and become very hard and sore to touch. This can take days to settle back down.

My remedy is total avoidance of these triggers as best I can and rest in a clean air environment.

Trigger Denial or Unaware?

I had trigger denial and then chose to face the facts. I didn't want to believe that my dogs could be causing me trouble breathing, so I looked at everything else around them. Still I was having difficulties, so I did some experiments and changed things (see under Pets) and that reduced and at times eliminated my breathing issues when they were close to me. *Below are my two fur girls Cleo 9yr and Vee 15yr RIP.*

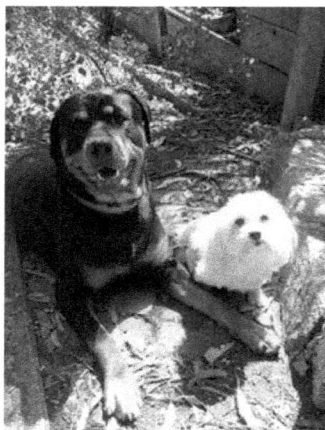

When I have conducted home inspections via online programs for people with RADS, they are unaware of the impact various everyday items can have on their breathing. I am also aware many products can be overlooked because sometimes the smell or fume from one trigger can *overlap* with another trigger, making it difficult to identify each culprit, so in some cases people need assistance.

Some triggers can be right there in your home or workplace and have a huge impact on your breathing and you may be unaware because you have done a particular task over and over pre RADS and never had an issue before.

An example could be, you go into the shed to get a tool and moments later you have trouble breathing. You are unaware it's the petrol in the lawnmower or the grease on the tools that were the trigger and you don't join the dots because you went in and out for years prior to getting RADS, without any issue. I ask people who contact me, to go through their daily routine and it's not uncommon for them to be using products or doing some task in or out the home, that cause them to have trouble breathing and they are totally unaware. It's often simple everyday items that are easily changed or removed once they are made aware of it. I was in the same loop when I first got RADS and had no idea I was contaminating myself and causing so many breathing issues but once I finally identified, changed or removed them, my breathing difficulties ceased or became less.

When travelling, I was unaware how dramatically location and climate impacted on my breathing, so now I do my best to avoid extreme temperatures and humidity. The degree of respiratory distress I had when in a humid climate was a surprise to me and as soon as I travelled to a different location away from that element, my breathing dramatically improved.

When I am in a safe clean air environment with no triggers, I feel good and do not have any breathing problems and no pain in my lungs and that is how I should feel (save for any other health issues aside from RADS). I often hear so much joy and relief in people's voices when they share feeling the same way, so it's comforting knowing others with this condition, can have such a positive experience too, when in a safe clean air environment.

Are My Breathing Issues All in My Head?

For me, the short answer is no! Flatly no! I mean seriously, who would want to live like this? Since having RADS, the breathing issues I experience have always been from an exposure to a trigger of some kind. That's a "physical" reaction brought about from inhaling a "physical" trigger.

I am aware there are some non-medical conditions that a heightened emotional state or exercise etc. can cause difficulty breathing or some form of respiratory distress however that is *not* my experience with my breathing issues.

When I was injured, living alone experiencing multiple triggers was exhausting and frightening not understanding why it was happening and having to phone for ambulance support on too many occasions.

Due to the onslaught of life-threatening breathing issues and suffocation I was experiencing, I became extremely anxious and started having panic attacks. I can't put into words how terrifying this felt and I knew I had to do something about it. I realized my anxiety, stress and panic attacks were *prolonging* my breathing issues, however they were **not** the reason they started.

It took months for me to devise ways to learn and manage my anxiety and stress during a breathing issue and in turn my panic attacks eventually subsided.

My work injury, employment, insurance, work-cover and litigation stress was enough to send me into the depths of depression as it was a very difficult time for me dealing with all these situations alone. At times I would feel bewildered, upset and extremely angry at the thoughtless acts or conditions I had to endure.

Years later I took some comfort in speaking to other people from around the world with RADS also going through and facing similar situations.

In regard to employment, I believe no-one should go to work and be left with a lifelong illness or condition.

Isolation

Another very difficult fall out from RADS, was the self-imposed isolation, as it was easier that way because so many people I came into contact with caused me various levels of breathing difficulties. I was amazed that I could smell the spray tan on their skin, the soap they used to shower with or the conditioner in their hair.

Perfume and aftershave were my arch enemies and I became hypervigilant, anxious and frightened because with one sniff, my airways could react so severely, I could start to suffocate. It was frightening and also lonely because no-one seemed to understand that I went to work feeling good and then left with an injury to my airway and lung and now I was super sensitive to all kinds of smells rendering me breathless or gasping for air. My whole world changed from ONE breath and it was traumatizing and confusing. I was calling for an ambulance on a weekly basis and felt uncomfortable doing this, as I had never had to call them before and I was confused not understanding why this was happening.

After or during a breathing issue sometimes friends or work colleagues would suggest, *"why don't you inhale a puffer"* or *"maybe it's just allergies"* or *"don't sensitivities give you a headache?"* I would feel frustrated, upset and annoyed because to me, they had no understanding or comprehension as to the level of seriousness my breathing issues were causing me. They weren't able to see or feel the extent of trauma and physical pain each attack was having on me. They could be life-threatening, debilitating, exhausting and very draining so instead of trying to explain, I would close down the conversation and back away.

At times there was no warning, a trigger may not have a smell and I would start to feel my airways restricting, like I was being choked from the inside out. On one occasion I ended up back in hospital and had the triage nurse cause me more problems breathing due to her perfume and then I had a doctor walk toward me wearing strong aftershave, so out of fear and desperation I began yelling at him to keep away because I could smell him from down the hallway and my airways began closing. After that incident, I did all I could to not end up in hospital.

Prior to my injury, I loved working and enjoyed being a people person and getting out and about. Having RADS, I now saw my friends pull away because I was just "too hard" to be around because I seemed to have breathing issues at the most random times. I didn't understand, so how on earth could I expect anyone else to? I had to stop work and locked myself away to survive.

In my experience, this condition can be very anti-social because you have to put your health first and some people just "don't get it" and still wear scented products like fragrant deodorants or body lotions etc. and then I end up having to quickly back away from them, while they are looking at me as if I had lost my marbles. What's worse is when friends have gone to the trouble of not wearing perfume or aftershave but I can still smell fabric softener on their clothes. On many occasions I would have them sit across from me in the wind, so the breeze blew the smell away from me. It can be so arduous and testing on your friends and family.

After each breathing issue I became extremely worried my airways would not heal and I would be left in a state of breathlessness. I would cry myself to sleep and had nightmares about it and was so grateful I would survive a night and my body would eventually heal, until the next onslaught.

It felt like anytime I stepped out my front door I was presented with a myriad of odours that were potentially life-threatening to me, so I stayed inside a lot and my friendship circle dwindled down to a catch up every few months with one cousin and one friend who were both considerate in accommodating my airway sensitivities.

Days turned into weeks and weeks turned into months and before I knew it, two and a half years had passed. During this time, I reached out to a doctor in the UK because she was the only person I could find at that time, who was researching and publishing work on RADS. She kindly responded and was very supportive and we shared some emails back and forth and I updated her with my progress. I was relentlessly, trialing and testing countless methods to decrease my triggers. It was exhausting and at times scary and eventually I had success and implemented one at a time. I practiced these new strategies and my Plan of Action over and over. These new tools also assisted me to cope more calmly with my breathing issues and while it was now automatic and proved positive and successful, it was a work in progress as I was faced with new triggers on a daily or weekly basis.

To help combat my isolation, I made a short video on YouTube® hoping someone else in the world with RADS might reach out. I also taught myself how to build a website, one to document some of my private journey living with this unique condition and the other as an information resource about RADS compiling material from my personal research and that from medical professionals. This all took a long time to achieve due to my health being so unpredictable however I was really proud of the outcome and hoped it was helpful and useful information.

I was now heading toward my third year living with RADS and I was still isolated and feeling very lonely and depressed and then it happened! I started to receive emails from all over the world. I vividly remember my first contact and it was a very emotional and heartfelt time for us both. It was wonderful and uplifting to know I was not alone and others mirrored the same struggles and reactions from triggers living with RADS.

Over the years to follow, people contacted me and each were at different stages, some only starting their new journey, while others had lived with RADS for decades and I found them to be so courageous and inspiring.

This motivated me to create a Facebook Group so those with RADS could have a place to chat and share their journey and know they are not alone. I am proud (yet sad) to say there are over one hundred people in the group from all over the world. Check RADS International under Facebook Groups.

It's hard to maintain friendships when you have RADS and even harder to find new friends. I can't stress enough how important it is to have mental health support, speaking to a Psychologist, counsellor, mentor or even just someone kind and understanding to have regular chats with about how you are feeling.

Some ideas for things to do if you are in isolation and feeling well enough:-

Write your life story - create a fictional story - write poetry - write a song – write a blog – read a book - learn a new skill online - learn a new language – try cooking a new recipe – re-organize your cupboards – clean out your wardrobe – detox each room from chemicals - research a subject you are passionate about - draw (with non-toxic colour pens, felt pens etc.) - paint (with non-toxic paint) – watch movies – write a movie –learn about a subject that interests you - build something - learn a song – make a video - play cards – play board games – do a puzzle – get a pet – learn some new breathing techniques - call a friend – be a support to someone.

SUPPORT

Family and Friends

When I was injured, I felt, fear, terror, anger, shock, grief, and loss. It took me some time to comprehend what had happened because the breathing issues I experienced were so intense and it turned my life upside down. I realize how important it would have been to have had an information or a guidance type book, to help me navigate my new life and my triggers with family and friends and to support me in learning "how" to live with RADS in and outside my home. Also encouraging friends and family to embrace new rules to manage, limit or remove triggers, would be a Win-Win!

Doing simple things like **not** wearing perfume, aftershave, scented products, burn candles, **not** using air fragrances, scented fabric softener, scented toilet products, chemicals and scented cleaning products etc. There are many other suggestions listed throughout my book which I hope you find useful.

A wonderful doctor once said to me "Having an injury like RADS that is under your skin makes it very challenging for people to understand just how very serious it can be. If people could see your injury, I'm sure they would be a lot kinder." How very true.

If you have family and friends offer kindness, compassion, patience and understanding to help while you learn and navigate a new way to live, then that's wonderful and very supportive.

To follow are just some of the ways my family and friends have been kind and considerate over the years in accommodating my sensitivities: -

- Check with me if they smell ok before hugging hello
- Not wearing scented/fragrant products when they are around me
- Put away all their potentially triggering household items if I visit
- If I stayed, cleaned out a spare room to assist my triggers
- Move far away from me if smoking outside
- Wear the plastic cape if they feel they might be wearing something that could smell
- Cleaned their whole house and bathroom with vinegar the night before I came to visit
- Especially meet up with me at places near the beach, so I could get lots of ocean air
- Don't shower before visiting me, just in case their soap or body wash triggers me
- Keep a change of tops in their car in the event what they are wearing triggers me
- Changed their washing liquids so their clothes wouldn't smell of fragrance
- One friend even built an outside shower for me to use when I was visiting, just in case their inside bathroom gave me triggers. OMG how great was that!

Please understand the above didn't happen overnight and for some changes, it has taken years to work with my new life rules and I really appreciate it when my family and friends remember.

If they do forget, they usually feel worse than me and I have my Plan of Action to minimize exposures, so I work through it without panic or stress.

Change can be difficult for some family and friends and having RADS means change needs to happen quickly to slow down, limit or stop breathing issues. Having patience and understanding while both parties learn the new rules is really helpful.

There are people with RADS who don't have support from family or loved ones due to a myriad of reasons and this can place them in extremely difficult situations.

If this has happened to you then I'm very sorry and encourage you to speak to your doctor or medical professional and seek guidance and support.

Legal Team

If you have been injured at work or injured as a result in other circumstances, then you may need to speak to a lawyer to determine if you have a case. Finding a law firm who has experience with RADS or respiratory related issues is extremely helpful. I also found it useful, while it was fresh in my mind to write or email myself details about how my exposure happened, the events leading up to it and if there were any witnesses etc. Just trying to live with RADS and how unpredictable it can be, is hard enough, let alone trying to navigate through the legal system, so finding a good legal team and be guided by them is important. If you are going through litigation and you are using social media, it may be useful to let your legal team know.

If you are a legal company who is familiar with Workcover and cases of toxic exposure or alike, then please email your details for our database. radsinternational@gmail.com Thank you

Medical Professionals: - General Practitioner

Having a GP who is close by and understands the uniqueness of RADS is extremely helpful. After I was diagnosed, I went in search for a local GP who listened and I found a great doctor who was not only a good support, she also knew the WorkCover system and that was an enormous help.

After I explained how much better I felt when I was near the ocean and sea air, she strongly suggested I move and with her encouragement I did and it's been the best thing I did! Due to relocating, I had to go in search for a new GP and finally struck gold when I found a wonderful local Doctor who fully understood my RADS and he provides unwavering support to this day, so I'm extremely fortunate!

Medical Professionals:- Lung - Respiratory Specialists – Pulmonologist

If you have already been diagnosed with RADS, then you may already have a Respiratory Specialist or Pulmonologist supporting you and if so that's great. If you found them to be helpful, supportive and knowledgeable about RADS, then I encourage you to email their details for our database of medical professionals familiar with this unique condition.

If you are a medical professional reading this and you are familiar with RADS, please do the same. Email radsinternational@gmail.com thank you.

Sadly, many people who contact me have trouble finding a specialist in their town or city. So, I suggest you could try calling a large hospital and ask if they have a Respiratory/Lung Department (or similar) and if not, ask which hospital closest to you does have one? You may find you have to travel a fair distance, as I know people have travelled interstate. Once you do find one, it might be worth asking if any of the specialists are familiar with RADS.

If you are still having trouble finding someone, then you are welcome to email me and I can check our database.

It took me some time to find my Respiratory Specialist. He has been a wonderful pillar of calm and sound medical advice and remains in contact since diagnosing me with RADS in 2013. He professionally navigated our WorkCover system, which was arduous to say the least, providing copious reports needed for my legal team. It's been a long road and I am grateful to him for his ongoing support, time and kindness in being accommodating of my sensitivities.

Please keep in mind, if you are going down the road of litigation or workers compensation it is imperative to have a medical professional who is willing to follow through with all the medical reports that will be needed throughout your litigation.

Medical Professionals:- Psychologist

Finding a psychologist who is familiar with respiratory issues and the Work-Cover system is extremely helpful. If you are going through litigation or have been through it, then you understand how very stressful that is, let alone living with RADS, so mental health support is paramount. I was most fortunate to be referred to a wonderful psychologist, who also has extensive knowledge with work-related injuries and has been a great support since my diagnosis.

Positive Peers

I do my best to share my time and energy with people who are supportive, proactive, open to new ideas and we learn from each other. They are RADS Warriors who are courageous in trying different strategies to help themselves and improve their life living with reactive airways.

RADS can be a very difficult condition to live with, unique from other conditions and when you are isolated it can be hard to maintain a positive outlook.

That's when peers who also have RADS are great to chat to as they know first-hand the different levels of breathing issues that can be experienced. Having support and doing our best to have a "Can Do" attitude inspires me to strive for the stars!

Suicidal thoughts?

In my case anger, fear and frustration were at the forefront of my thoughts and I felt fragile and very reactive if people minimized my situation.

Just staying alive felt exhausting!

RADS can be so life-changing and people may need extra support. So, if you are not coping, then I strongly encourage you to please seek out a mental health professional, speak to your doctor or call Lifeline or a similar service in your country or call emergency.

Some numbers for Lifeline are below and you can find many more on the internet for your country.

Australia	Lifeline	13 11 14
Australia	Veterans After Hours Crisis Counselling	1800 011 046
Australia	Beyond Blue	1300 22 4636
Australia	National Emergency	000

USA	National Suicide Prevention Lifeline	1-800-273-8255
USA	The Veterans Crisis Line	1-800-273-8255
USA	The Trevor Lifeline	1-866-488-7386
USA	National Emergency	911

New Zealand	Lifeline Aotearoa- within Auckland	09-5222999
New Zealand	for those outside Auckland	0800 543 354
New Zealand	need to talk?	1737
New Zealand	National Emergency	111

Canada	Crisis Services Canada	1-833-456-4566
Canada	National Emergency	911

United Kingdom	Samaritans	116 123 999
United Kingdom	National Emergency	112

The above numbers were correct as at March 2020

Superannuation – Total Permanent Disability (TPD) Claim

In Australia, if you have been diagnosed with RADS and you have Superannuation, your fund may offer Total Permanent Disability (TPD) and you may be eligible for a lump sum claim. So, it's a good idea to call your Superannuation Company and check and if you are eligible, they can guide you through their procedure. Prepare yourself for needing reports from your doctor and specialist. I also believe some law firms can do the same thing for you, for a fee. Superannuation may be different in each country, so it may be worth a call and check with yours.

I have always had a strong moral conscience and appreciate a company who has a high level of workplace safety, so when companies put profit before people's safety, that makes me angry. I feel my work injury was totally avoidable, so this incited feelings of resentment and anger and I lost all trust in the company and humanity.

It felt like each day I woke up, I was living in some parallel universe and it was all a bad dream. I feel I was in shock and experienced trauma and was grieving the life I had. I was alone, confused and angry and life as I knew it had gone and I was left with this new life of over analysing each breath I took, for fear it would cause my airways to react and I would suffocate.

Not only was I left with serious breathing issues, doctors seemed to fail in understanding how bad they were. I lived alone, I had no moral support and no sick leave left, so no income and trying to cope with the WorkCover, insurance and legal systems, my life was a mess and my mindset was not in a good place and I don't blame me! That time of my life was horrible and after speaking to other people with RADS, I know I'm not the only person who has gone through similar struggles.

My rage was kept alive and well oiled due to many years of litigation. Having to recall every detail, step and moment of how I got injured and convey the immense impact that living with RADS now had on my everyday life, was draining and exhausting. I was sick of hearing myself talk about it but I had to invest energy in each conversation to the all-important "listeners" who held my financial life in their hands. Having to immerse myself energetically with each conversation was gruelling because I was very sick. Also being judged and assessed at every step was soul-destroying. I hated the whole system and I loathed those before me who had lied about an injury because I felt they had carved this horrid path of suspicion and scepticism I was now having to endure and, in my mind, that was totally unfair because my injury was real!

Just staying alive and breathing was now at the top of my list!

No medications I tried seemed to be working and there were no discussions about other treatments or therapies to help reduce my breathing issues. The longer this went on, the more depressed and hopeless I felt until one night I had a serious chat to myself; *"Surely this can't be it? There's no medication that can help, **nothing**? Ok, so if there's nothing out there to help me, **then game on!** I'm going to have to do it myself! There is **NO WAY** I am going to sit back and do nothing, **that is not going to happen!"**

I was blown away that in this big wide world there was nothing to help me live with my RADS! No tablet, no quick fix, no steps to take, no direction, no book, no information, zip, nothing! My mindset took a big shift from desperate and hopeless to getting all fired up determined and driven! I wanted to live and not just *exist* in life, regardless of having these extreme sensitivities, so I made a choice to fight like a Warrior and no longer live in fear and that's when the term **RADS Warrior** was born!

I remember laughing to myself as images popped into my head. Me, a fifty plus chick, all the way down here in Australia in a warrior's outfit swinging a sword going into battle but that's exactly how I felt. It was a battle, every day was a battle and I could either sit in the trenches alone or make a plan and forge ahead. I was going to give it my best shot and I was determined to make a positive difference.

First, I had to take control of my own health because it was abundantly clear there was no help out there. I decided to harness my brainpower and skill-set and put it to good use creating different methods and strategies to manage my breathing issues and reduce or eliminate triggers. I used myself as a guinea pig and this took time, commitment, patience and courage because sometimes things I tried didn't go to plan and left me in life-threatening situations.

Over time as new methods proved successful, they became part of my RADS Tool Kit or Plan of Action, forming the vital tools I use to manage my breathing issues and reduce or eliminate triggers. I practiced them over and over vigilantly every day. I also implemented and practiced new strategies and other therapies to rebuild my mental health and boost my confidence and this was crucial and important work. I created new directives in my mind that would slingshot over to solutions which kept me safe.

Doing work on yourself takes time, commitment and lots of practice and having someone to speak to along the way, who is positive and supports the work you are doing is very helpful. For me, my psychologist was encouraging and someone I could trust and share my thoughts and feelings as I began my new life journey.

I was now on a mission and very passionate about promoting awareness about RADS and sharing the successful strategies and methods that worked for me, in the hope it helped others. My mindset was now in a much healthier place and I was ready for the battle ahead!

Disability

To be perfectly honest, when my specialist first uttered my name and the word "disability" in the same sentence I had a total meltdown. This took me by surprise, so having my psychologist was helpful in airing all my thoughts and feelings in relation to this.

I decided to make a deal with myself, that anytime anyone used the word disability in reference to my RADS, I would swap it for **"Super Power".** Due to the fact I now had an extremely heightened sense of smell, when needed; my **Super Power** would keep me safe. So, I was now a **RADS Warrior** with a **Super Power**! How cool is that!

CREATE A SAFE ROOM or
FIND A SAFE BREATHING PLACE

I share my following experiences with you to highlight ***never giving up***! I feel sure someone out there will be reading this who may have had, or is having a similar journey. Well, maybe not similar but maybe situations where things just didn't go as well as planned or hoped. ***So again... never give up***!

After getting RADS I had countless breathing issues in my home, so out of desperation I had to create a sterile room to allow me to breathe normally, commonly known as a "safe room". This was not an easy feat and took many weeks to realize. I decided my en-suite bathroom would be the best room, as it had mostly tiled floors and walls and I could empty it out easily. Well, so I thought!

I put on a mask and gloves (old ones as new rubber gloves cause me breathing issues) and noticed the strong smell of perfume was still in my bathroom cupboard even though I cleaned it out with hot water. I decided to roll up two old towels and pushed them inside the cupboards and then taped the doors shut. I hoped the old towels would absorb the smells and it seemed to work. I wiped down all the floor and wall tiles with hot water and it was now very clean and as sterile as I could make it. I set up pillows and comforters on the floor as a place to sleep while I was trying to work out what else in my home was triggering me.

Unfortunately doing all this and not having a good mask, I had contaminated myself with fumes and dust and was now experiencing great pain in my lung, so it was very uncomfortable when I tried to lay down. The air in my bathroom seemed ok so I persisted for a few nights but my lung was still extremely sore and I began feeling desperate to get out of my home and get anywhere that had clean air.

Staying at friends' homes was not an option because of the various chemicals I could detect, however one friend who lived fifteen minutes from the Surf Coast, suggested I could sleep in my tent in his yard. I had driven the two hour journey to the Great Ocean Road and Surf Coast the week before and was thrilled to find the pristine strong winds blowing in from the Antarctic and the salty air was absolutely wonderful and so healing for my lungs. I had travelled to many beaches over the previous months in search of the best air I could find in Victoria to heal the tenderness in my lungs and this was the best I found. It was still close by to amenities and a large hospital not too far, so it ticked a lot of boxes for me.

I packed my little tent, air mattress, sleeping bag and deck chair and headed off on the long drive. Once I was all set up in my friend's backyard, I climbed inside the tent and immediately the smell from the plastic mattress was coming through the cover I had over it and that caused me more breathing issues, so I quickly opened the vents on the little tent but it was no good. I was now feeling extremely unwell and had to get out. I tried to sleep in my car but my lung was hurting and it was very uncomfortable, so I packed up and drove fifteen minutes down to the beach. I parked as close to the crashing waves as I could but you are not allowed to sleep in your car or camp at these beaches. So, I took out my deck chair and sleeping bag and set it up right next to the ocean and wrapped myself in my sleeping bag and sat there under the stars.

I can't describe how wonderful it was to have that clean salt air billowing toward me and with each careful breath I felt the inflammation in my lung slowly easing and my airways settling. Finally, some relief! As it approached midnight, I started to get cold and frightened as I was alone and every noise seemed to be magnified. There was a toilet block close to the ocean and I knew the breeze blew under and over the doors and it was clean and they had sturdy locking doors. So very desperate to continue getting that healing ocean air, I grabbed my deck chair and sleeping bag and set it up in the last stall closest to the ocean and locked myself in.

As I sat there with my sleeping bag wrapped around me, I began quietly sobbing. I was sobbing because I couldn't believe I was actually sitting in a chair in a toilet and that I was so grateful the stall didn't stink of urine or chemicals. Through tears of exhaustion and tiredness, I also thought how very sad that this is what my life had been reduced to. Who would have believed it? All from ONE breath!

Over the next few hours, I tried to quietly focus my thoughts on the fact I was safe, albeit a bit cold but my breathing was improving and the pain in my lung was softening and that's all that mattered.

Knowing how very good I felt each time I was inhaling that amazing ocean air, I made a big decision for my health and wellbeing. I decided to move from suburbia, sell my home and buy a block of land as close to the ocean as I could afford and build the best RADS friendly home I could. This was a massive decision but I had to do it for my health. I wanted access to that amazing ocean air anytime and didn't want to have to drive a four to five hour round trip to get it and I never wanted to be in this situation ever again!

For the next few months, I travelled that long highway every weekend and each time, that pristine salt air would heal my aching lung and calm my airways. I knew I had made the right decision, so I started to look for a room to rent. (check: Looking for accommodation) I put great thought into the design of my new home so it would be a safe haven in the event there was ever a fire nearby and I did as much research as I could in regard to having the least toxic building products used. Even doing all this, it's now close to four years since building finished and although I can now be inside my home for periods of time, I'm still not able to sleep inside at night without experiencing lung pain the next day or spiting up blood.

I did think about selling but then, I wouldn't be sure what I was buying, so I am trying to just wait it out as I am determined and my goal is to eventually sleep inside. Whatever chemical or toxin is causing me the pain in my lung is getting less and less each month and year but it's a slow process and in spite of the money I have spent in changing paints, floor coverings and having expensive air quality tests done, I'm yet to identify and remove the culprit. That is why I purchased a campervan and have been sleeping in it, in my driveway for the past four years and sometimes I will drive and sleep close to the ocean or go on road trips and follow the coast always seeking out that healing salt air.

So you would think that's the end of that right .. but no **there's more!**

As a stroke of bad luck, the battery under the bed in my campervan leaked copious sulphur while I was sleeping in my van in my driveway and the concentration of fumes could have killed me if not for waking up and using some of my oxygen in my small tank. I thought there was a gas leak *outside*, so I shut the roof air hatch not realizing it was coming from **inside** my van under my bed!

The smell and my breathing became so bad I had to exit the van and go inside my home for safety and it was so serious the fire brigade were called. I was now no longer able to sleep in my van, drive it or go near it for weeks due to the sulphur smell leaching into the rubber, plastic and cabinetry work. It had to be written off and that took months!

I was now in a bad situation with nowhere safe to sleep, so I decided to purchase an outside daybed to try to sleep out on that on my back patio at night. I tried airing it out for a few days but I immediately had breathing issues when I tried to sleep on it due to the strong chemical smell coming from the canopy and mattress covers. I used blankets and towels to smother the mattress and canopy cover but then I got bitten by mozzies through the night. So, I made a mosquito net that covered the front of the daybed and thought I would be ok.

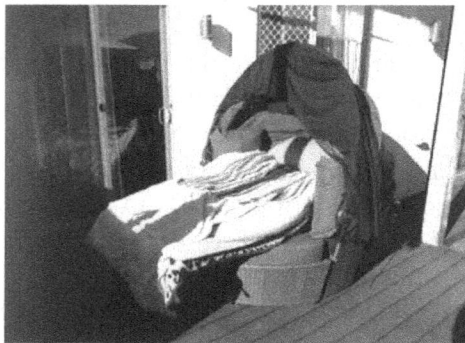

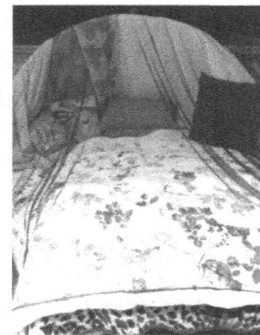

Finally, somewhere safe to sleep where I could breathe! It worked well for the next few weeks and my lungs and airways were slowly healing and I could drive to the beach most days in a small rental car (see under Rental cars) so that was a huge help.

Then late one night as I was fast asleep outside on my daybed, I woke to cracking thunder and the most ferocious storms and pelting rain. I can remember laughing at the irony of it all, as I ran around in my nightie at 2am madly trying to pull the bed apart and put the cover on to protect it from the rain. The whole daybed was being blown across my small patio and I was getting absolutely drenched with rain. I felt like I was living in some dark comedy movie!

I moved all the bedding inside and dried off. I then thought I could set up a bed inside my large shower area but I only lasted a short time due to the strong smell of mortar between the tiles and I was very fearful I might kick my leg out through the night and smash the shower screen. I then moved myself into my lounge area as it was the largest room in the house. I was now exhausted and pushed my two-seater recliner sofa close to my back-sliding doors and opened them to allow the chilled cold air to blow in and thought I would be ok. I was, until I went to sleep and forgot where I was and rolled off and fell onto my concrete floor waking up wondering where I was and why I was so cold.

Seriously, again I had to laugh because if I didn't, I would have cried as this was one bad event after another and you just couldn't make this stuff up!

After waiting four months to get the ok from the insurance company to get a replacement van, I then had to wait another six weeks for the new van to off-gas and then I was able to sleep in it, in my driveway again. The insurance company had no comprehension of the predicament I was in, just trying to find or create a safe place to sleep and how very sick it was making me each time I tried to sleep inside.

After speaking to many people with RADS, I know mine isn't an isolated situation as trying to find or create a safe place to sleep is so very important and we have to do whatever is needed to breathe!

Anyhow, back to safe rooms and places and some useful and positive information to follow!

Creating a safe room, space or place where you can breathe without any triggers is extremely important and below, I share with you what I have done in the past that worked really well when I was renting a room, while my home was being built.

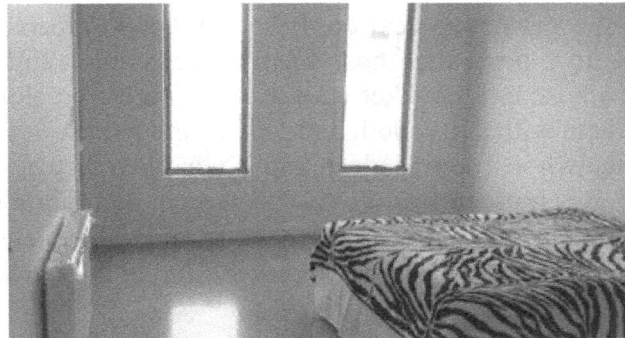

The Room

Firstly, if you can get someone to do the following then that is a massive help. The first thing is to pick a room that is going to become your "safe room." If you are doing this alone, then I suggest you put on a good quality mask (maybe one that has a carbon active filter) and if you have overalls or a dust coat or an old sweater and pants and cover your hair too. A shower cap or scarf could do the trick and some gloves and goggles or eye protection. Dust can be a very serious trigger, so it really is worth investing the time to put all this protective gear on.

Clean out the room of absolutely everything, including the curtains and when you take down curtains, do it slowly and be mindful they can hold a lot of fine dust. Also carefully take the window screens out and if you can take them outside don't bang them around as they usually contain a lot of fine dust and just leave them outside for now. If you can't remove the window screens then that's ok and do the following.

Once the room is empty get a damp cloth and <u>slowly</u> wipe down all the walls, curtain tracks, door and any inbuilt cupboards etc. Then if the screens are still in the windows, with a clean damp warm cloth, start at the <u>top</u> of the screen and wipe in a slow downward motion <u>once</u> and then rinse the cloth of dirt in the warm water, squeeze it out and repeat. Keep wiping in a downward motion once, until you have wiped the whole screen and there is no more dust on the cloth. Then wipe in an upward motion <u>once</u> and repeat. Don't get impatient and wipe up and down as it may fluff up fine dust.

Once the screen has been cleaned, wipe the inside window frame with a warm cloth and then the skirting boards. Then last is the floor (obviously if it's not carpet) mop it with a damp cloth. If it is carpet then ask someone else to vacuum it or ensure you have your protective gear on to do it. Once that's done, then go outside and dust yourself off because fine dust may have fallen on you.

If you feel uncomfortable or have any breathing issues whatsoever doing any of the above, then IMMEDIATELY STOP and do not begin cleaning until your breathing is good or get someone else to do it. Be sensible and if need be, do it in stages or a little bit at a time and ensure you wear your protective gear.

With your protective gear on, if your window screens are outside and you have access to a hose, then hose them down without fluffing up dust. If you don't have a hose use a bucket with warm water and a cloth to clean them and then wipe them with a dry cloth and replace them back in the room.

Once the whole room is clean and if you have carpet, get some fresh clean non-smelly (i.e. no scents of washing detergent and fabric softener) sheets and lay them over the carpet to smother it. If you don't have enough sheets to cover a whole room, then ensure you smother the carpet around where you would get out of bed.

Once all the cleaning was done, then I sat in the room for as long as I needed to test the air and concentrate on how my breathing "felt". If I had a breathing issue or a reaction then I may need to investigate other factors like, what other rooms are close by or what might be blowing through the window into the room from outside or if the room was recently painted etc.

It's important to be mindful of where your safe room is in the home. If it is positioned right next to a bathroom where people are using scented products these may waft into your safe room, or if it is nearby to the laundry room. If this was the case then I would hang a big towel or even a sheet across the whole door frame and put a rolled-up towel at the base of my door to help stop fumes coming under the closed door.

If you have a window in your bedroom that is near a busy street, then be mindful about fumes or pollution blowing through. In my previous home, my window was only open a few centimetres and the fumes of diesel from minimal traffic would filter in and cause me breathing difficulties.

The Super Powers of RADS are quite remarkable!

I also had to cut back bushes growing outside my window as some omitted a scent that gave me breathing issues.

It's very important to check inside your home for any gas leaks and outside your home for gas or sewer pipes that could be leaking and omitting a fume. If this is the case then immediately leave and call the gas company. Again, if you have any breathing difficulties then it would be sensible to go straight to hospital.

After sitting in my empty room and not having any reactions, I started to bring in ONE item at a time. First was my bed frame and I put it on the floor and sat in the room with the door shut and concentrated on how my breathing felt. Due to having no reaction I set it up. Then I repeated the process bringing in ONE item at a time like bed slats (some new pine slats or other timbers may cause breathing issues), my mattress (some mattresses could have formaldehyde on them and this could cause breathing issues), side tables (if timber, then check what the table is made from and if it has any mould on it or inside as mould could cause breathing issues) drawers (if timber then check what the drawers are made from and if it has any mould on it or inside as mould could cause breathing issues) and slowly I would test how I felt with each item in the room.

You may not be able to hang old washed curtains back up due to entrenched smells, so you may need to invest in new curtains. I purchased some curtains that were all cotton (with no block out) and I hand washed them, hung them outside to dry and then hung them in the room and had no reaction to them. I hope you find curtains that don't cause you any breathing issues. You could also look into getting metal blinds, which I had installed in one room. I just had to keep an eye on the dust they can catch and ensure they were cleaned regularly.

Also, be mindful of the clothes, towels, sheets etc. you bring into the room. If they have been washed in a scented or chemical product, they may cause breathing issues. (see under Laundry)

It's a process of elimination and proved to be successful for me when renting a room in a home I lived at while building my new house. I feel the key is to not rush and take your time while you assess each item you bring into the room. Notice how your body reacts or feels and hopefully it won't react and you can create your safe room.

It's important to note that due to everyday life, doors and windows being opened, people coming in etc. safe rooms can sometimes be compromised. When this has happened to me, I put on a good mask, air my room out, run my air purifier (see under air purifiers), put on the overhead fan and fluff my curtains to help release any fumes or dust that may have invaded my safe room. If I experience any breathing issues, I will go to the beach and lay in my van to heal until I am able to go back to my safe room.

I hope the above suggestions are helpful and useful to you.

Vehicle – Another safe place could be a vehicle. If it has no inside smells that trigger you then that's good and if it has room to lay down and stretch out, that would be helpful. My car didn't trigger me which was great but it wasn't a practical model for me to sleep in.

Campervan/Motorhome – As long as there are no triggers inside, these vehicles can be a useful safe place and can usually be quickly and easily moved if the environment changes and that's very helpful. They can also be used to sleep in if visiting friends' or family and in place of staying in motels if you are away on holidays or travelling.

Caravan – Another safe space can be caravans. As long as there is nothing inside that triggers you, then they can be a good safe place. Although some are permanent and cannot be moved, others can be and that's helpful if the environment changes and you need to move. They can also be used to sleep in if visiting friends' or family and in place of staying in motels if you are away on holidays or travelling.

Chewing Gum

Who would have thought that something as simple as chewing gum could help? Allow me to explain a theory that was shared with me. When chewing gum, we create saliva and if there are fine dust particles or fumes in the air and they go into our mouth, then some may get caught in the saliva and we swallow it rather than inhale it.

Made sense to me and when I tried it, it worked! So, when I am out, or driving I am often chewing gum either with or without my mask on. I also find it helps to keep my throat saturated and I try to buy gum that has nothing artificial with all natural ingredients. Some people can't chew gum so they tell me they suck on different lozenges instead. I expect finding a sugar free one would be helpful.

Handheld Fan

I purchased a few inexpensive small hand fans online and they have been good if I go out where there are people close to me who maybe wearing fragrances that are a bother to me, so I just fan the smell away. Sometimes, I will use the fan to create the movement of air if I am in a place where the air is dense.

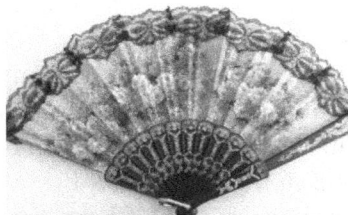

Masks

There are a number of masks on the market and I have tried many different ones over the years but none I have tried provide 100% protection from fumes or smoke. I am not currently able to wear the full respiratory type masks due to the smell of the latex or rubber face piece.

I have found the small 2 ply masks, commonly known as medical masks helpful in limiting some dust but useless in reducing or stopping fumes or smoke and they have a very short life span.

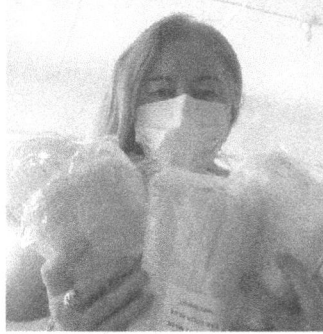

There are many different styles of masks on the market with some masks being made from a thick fabric with various charcoal filters and others are a simple cotton mask. When I am especially reactive, even the smell from a new small 2ply mask can give me breathing issues, so I will usually air them out before wearing them.

I also have some P2 masks and keep a couple in the glove box of my vehicle. The ones I have, come wrapped individually in their own plastic bag and I've never had any issue with them smelling. They are a lot thicker than the medical type masks and are quite large, so as to fit over all different size faces and each has an outlet valve. I might use the P2 masks if I have to use a public bathroom and they have been very helpful in reducing exposure to fragrances and other odors. Once used, I discard them in the bin,

Over the years I have tried various heavy duty masks with activated carbon or charcoal filters in them and although none filter out fumes by 100%, I have found one in particular to be very useful in helping me get through especially bad air situations like; high traffic, filling up my van at the fuel station, driving through road works, dust storms, pollution, some shopping centers and as needed. I have used this particular brand of mask for several years and tested it in various elements and in my opinion; it has worked very well in reducing my exposure to fumes, smoke and dust. If I am in an especially bad air situation in my vehicle, I will place my medical air tube under the chin of this mask and allow the air to envelop it, giving me a high percentage of clean air to breathe and time to get out of the area or away from the situation. My mask has removable filters in it, so I can change them and the outside is washable, so I can clean them after an exposure as the material can hold the smell.

I used to be self-conscious about wearing my mask but for me, the health benefits outweigh my vanity. These days there is a great selection of masks with great colors and designs, so depending on my mood I will change it around a bit.

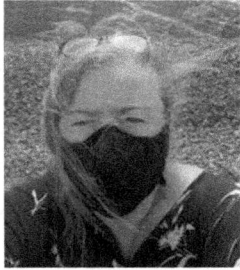

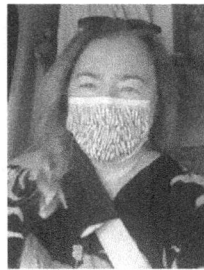

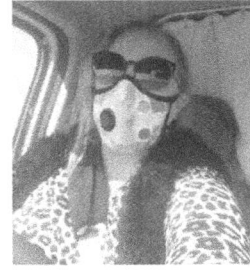

If I am having a good air day then I don't wear any masks and generally, I am wearing them less and less, now that I have reduced my triggers by way of living away from suburbia and pollutants.

It's very much a matter of trial and error until you find a mask that suits your specific needs. Changing or discarding your mask after it has absorbed a fume etc. is very important.

Someone once said to me, *"you'll be right you're wearing your mask,"* as I was boarding an open ferry. Wearing a mask does not mean I am "safe" from certain exposures. Fumes, smoke, vapor and sulphur could still penetrate my masks and cause serious breathing issues.

Medical Air / Oxygen

I was constantly calling paramedics due to my severe breathing problems and eventually worked out that when I was in a clean air environment, I felt good, so I went on a mission trying to figure out how to create that. I was regularly going to a nearby forest to just sit or walk around because when I was in certain parts of the forest, I could breathe well. After a big exposure, I would often get pain in my lung, so I would drive to the ocean at the Surf Coast, where I would lay in my car breathing in the clean salt air for hours or days. It did wonders for settling my airways, the pain in my lung and I could breathe so well when I was there.

So, I became very excited when I had my epiphany, which was life-changing for me and I share it with you.

The movement of clean air = dissipates a trigger and settles my airways

Just how would I create this? Then the penny dropped and I thought about the fact that oxygen is in a tank and that is "uncontaminated" by pollutants in the environment and when it's turned on, its moving air! I was eager and very excited to test my theory and when I did **IT WORKED** to calm my airways and settle my breathing and I was thrilled! I had been given oxygen for short periods by paramedics on many occasions, so I wanted to speak to my specialist to see if there were other products that could do the same.

You see, it *wasn't* that I *needed* oxygen to breathe because my pulmonary function tests had always been good, I just used the "uncontaminated moving clean air" part, to **help dissipate** a **trigger** and **calm my airways**, the same way it did at the beach and in the forest.

This is where I feel RADS is so unique, because based on my experience, when I am exposed to a trigger, my air-ways and vocal cords react **first** and my lung pain/reaction usually happens **after**. I don't ever recall having a lung issue *first* and *then* airway sensitivity.

When exposed to a trigger that leaves my airways sensitive, using medical air to calm my airways has been a great alternative if I'm unable to get to the beach and breathe the clean salt air.

I was so excited by the success of my trial, I contacted my Respiratory Specialist and the research doctor in the UK I had been corresponding with. Then with the support and guidance of my specialist, I logged my breathing issues for a period of time with a peak flow meter and a chart and had enough evidence to support him in prescribing what he felt would work best for me and that was a tank of **medical air** for home and a smaller tank (which is an oxygen tank, as I couldn't get medical air in a small tank) for in my vehicle.

No longer did I have to call paramedics or go to hospital. It gave me back some control and hope for a future that wasn't locked behind closed doors and the peace of mind I needed no matter if I was home or out. I use the small tank of oxygen in my vehicle for short periods to dissipate a trigger, when I am not travelling far or my large medical air tank for longer trips, if faced with compromising situations like, bitumen road works, smoke, dust storms, traffic fumes etc. and it's been a life-saver for me. It allows me autonomy to manage my own health and it's an integral part of my RADS Tool Kit.

Only on a couple of occasions, when I have been exposed to humidity or an unidentified trigger that I cannot smell or taste, I have experienced laboured breathing where my lung has felt heavy. At these times, my airways *did not* react *nor* were they sensitive. Gently using medical air at these times also helped me to recover.

It's been wonderful to connect with others living with RADS, who shared they were also prescribed medical air by their medical professionals and they've also had success. Speaking with your medical team about your health and specific situation is extremely important.

Medical Air / Oxygen – How I use it

Using the tank of medical air still left me with some challenges, due to the strong chemical smell of the plastic tubing and the plastic mask attached. I was fortunate to eventually find a used air hose, and purchased my own activated carbon material mask. When I'm away, I feed the tube under the chin of the mask so it rests on my chin near my mouth. I turn my tank on very low, so the air gently blows through the tube and circulates inside my mask and creates a mini "clean air environment" and works really well for me. I am very mindful of only using it for short periods.

Sometimes after a low trigger and if I am in a clean air environment, I just wave the tube near my mouth without the mask on and this allows me to gently breathe in the clean moving air and it has been very successful in also calming my airways and dissipating a trigger.

I am very careful to follow my specialist advice using my medical air or oxygen for limited periods when dissipating a trigger and that is usually from a minute or two and not more than about ten minutes.

When I am away travelling, I strap my large tank of medical air in the front of my van. If I am driving through extremely polluted or dusty terrain, I may put my mask on and have the tube feeding medical air inside my mask on very low, to help create a clean air environment inside my mask and to limit breathing in triggers. Again, I try to limit the time I use it.

Below shows me in my van with the prong tubing under the chin of my mask and the other is showing how I sometimes hold the tubing near my mouth to circulate the medical air and create moving clean air.

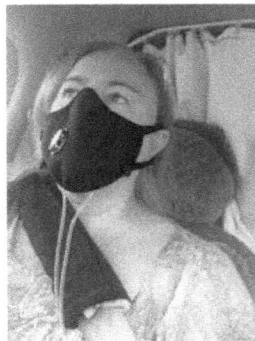

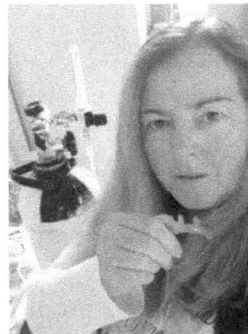

If after a trigger I have lung pain or my airways are still sensitive, I lay down in a clean air environment with an air purifier running and I may also wave the medical air tube near my mouth for a short time to get added clean air movement and it usually settles my airways. If there was a good sea breeze that day and I was well enough to make the short drive to the ocean, my first preference would be to go and sit or lay in my van at the beach and breathe in the salt air, which seems to be the fastest healing process for my lungs.

Tubing may have nose prongs and I do not put them in my nose because I don't like air blowing into my nose and up into my head, as I feel my sinuses are very sensitive. If I use the tube with prongs, I just feed the nose prong under the chin of my mask and rest it near my mouth (shown above) to circulate the medical air into my mask.

The whole purpose of the moving clean air is to dissipate the trigger and gently settle my airways down my throat.

You could cause serious harm to your health if you do not have medical consultation and supervision. This is extremely important, so always consult with your doctor or medical team. I have always followed the medical advice given to me when using my tanks of medical air or oxygen.

My small five kilo tank has a backpack which is helpful if I am going out walking however if it is a good air day then I might leave my tank in my vehicle and wear my mask or nothing at all, however I don't usually venture too far. Knowing I have my tank in my vehicle to use as needed if I get into a situation, gives me peace of mind and has saved me calling paramedics many times over the years.

My small tank is securely strapped in the front of my van between my two front seats. This way I can pull over, and quickly and easily access it as needed. I also carry a second small spare full tank of oxygen in the back of my van in the event my front tank is low or near empty and I just change them over if needed. The other larger tank of medical air is at home and I can move it around to different rooms and as mentioned, I will strap it in my van and take it with me, if I am going away on a longer trip.

Before any long trip, I always check where I can get a re-fill tank and fortunately there are many locations across Australia, which has been really helpful.

Medication

I am fortunate that aside from RADS my general health felt pretty good and prior to getting RADS my respiratory health felt fine. I had no allergies and was not aware of being sensitive to anything. When I am in a clean air environment my lung function has always felt pretty good and my tests post RADS are similar.

In the first 12 months of being injured, I was prescribed copious asthma inhalers with no success and some made my breathing worse, so this was very distressing. Eventually after being diagnosed with RADS, my specialist prescribed the steroid tablet Prednisolone and prior to creating my Plan of Action and reducing my triggers, I took it on a few occasions and have it on standby if ever needed.

For me, my "**go to**" is one or some of the following: -

- Heading to the ocean and breathing in clean salt air
- Walking or sitting in the forest in a great air spot
- Use my medical air
- Sitting near my air purifier in a safe room
  (i.e. a room that does not have anything in it that will trigger me)

I'm happy to say that since making changes in my life, identifying and reducing triggers implementing my Plan of Action, changing my mindset to a more positive mode, means I can manage my RADS without the need of any medication. Also, I've not gone to hospital for my breathing issues in years and I'm very happy about that!

To this day I continue to have consults with my Specialist and keep him updated with my progress and we discuss any new strategies I would like to try and he gives me his valued and important feedback and direction. This is <u>very</u> important as I am not a Doctor and he looks at things from a medical perspective and provides me with information and feedback I may not have thought about and need to consider for my specific situation, health and wellbeing. He has also kindly arranged my appointments via online programs for years, so I don't have to travel through the city to see him and be exposed to serious triggers, which is so helpful and appreciated.

It's been a journey of more than eight years of trial and error and a lot of time and personal research to identify reduce or eliminate my triggers and design methods to manage my breathing issues. This along with the movement of clean air is what I regard as pivotal, valuable and important information and what has successfully worked for my specific situation.

__Important Reminder__:- This book is written from my personal journey and is a guide and collation of suggestions only and not to be used by you in place of any medical professional or qualified and licensed professionals' instructions or medications that work for you. You should always consult your doctor when it comes to your personal health, or before you start any treatment.

Plastic Raincoat / Cape

I keep an "aired out" plastic raincoat cover at home for when a visitor might pop over. This is because sometimes people's clothes have fabric softener smell or the soap they used to shower with that morning can causing me breathing issues, so the plastic cape smothers the smell and stops it from lingering in my home. Cover and smother! My friends have been great by not being bothered if I have asked them to put it on before they come into my home.

It's so nice when people understand. *Below is my good friend Gail modelling the plastic cape I have at home.*

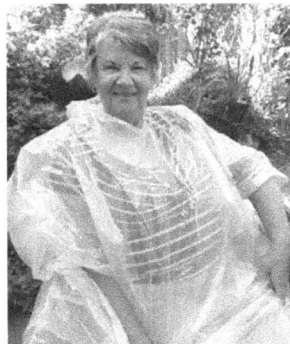

It's also been great for smothering strong deodorant smells when I have had tradies come into my home to do repairs and they have kindly put on the cape.

I have a plastic cape in my van ready to give any person travelling in my van who may be wearing perfume, or have used strong soap etc. So, it has come in very handy and stops their fragrant smell from transferring to the fabric seats in my van or on my furniture at home.

Once someone has worn it, I take it outside and put it on the line and hose it down to get the smell off the plastic and I leave it out to air for a few days, then it's ready to use again.

Steam Cup

Within days of my initial exposure part of my lung collapsed and I was so scared a memory popped into my head from when I was sixteen. I was babysitting a child who had croup and the mum said: "if he starts to cough or has any trouble breathing, turn the shower on and stand in the bathroom and let him gently breathe in some of the steam." So I did that, and I am convinced it saved my life because within moments I could feel the steam gently saturate my throat and enter my lung and slowly my airway relaxed and opened. I went out the next day and purchased a small handheld steamer cup and it became my most important possession while I was still figuring everything out.

I find steam to be a lovely gentle way to relax my airways, however too much or too hot can have a bad effect and cause serious injury, so I have always been very careful to get the temperature just right and just breathe in a very small amount at a time.

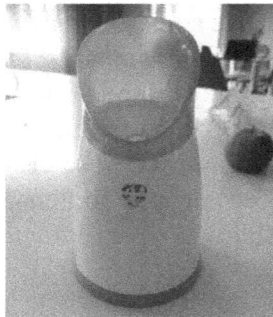

Water Bottle and Empty

With the amazing "Super Powers" of RADS I was able to smell and taste the chlorine and fluoride in my water at home. So, I purchased a ceramic water filter and it's now lovely and clean. I did purchase some bottled water when I was away and was surprised to find to me, it actually had a strange smell. If I ever buy bottled water again, I will always do a sniff test before drinking it.

I usually now take my own bottled water anywhere I go and I carry a small empty bottle, so if I happen to inhale a fume from people walking past me or near me, I stay calm and move away and gargle water from my water bottle and then discretely spit it into the empty bottle. I will do this about three or four times and it has helped me to dissipate the fume or trigger and helps to get rid of the taste. If I didn't do this after a strong exposure, I can wake up the next day and still have a strong smell and taste in my mouth and down my throat and sometimes a thin film of mucus.

I can also be left with sore lungs that can last a day or weeks depending on the severity of the exposure. I feel gargling and spitting out the contents immediately after an exposure has helped my recovery.

Regularly drinking clean water is also great because I find it helps to keep me hydrated and my throat saturated.

What Sooths My Throat and Clears Film in My Throat

I'm not a diabetic or on any special diet and have found sucking on a small piece of chocolate to be soothing down my throat or drinking a warm chocolate milk. It feels like it soothes and lines my throat with a silky film from the chocolate. I have also found a drink of warm lemon with some honey to be soothing or if you are on a special diet, then even just warm water can be soothing after a trigger.

Keeping my throat saturated by chewing gum has also been helpful or sucking on mild throat lozenge.

Some mornings when I have woken up with the smell and taste of the previous days trigger down my throat, I can also have what feels like a thin mucus film down my throat. To clear this, I might gargle with warm water and a pinch of pink salt or some salt water I have collected from the ocean and after a few gargles the film and foul taste is usually gone. When I was away travelling and had the same after effects from a trigger, the next day I had a few sips of a fizzy syrup soft drink and was surprised to find it seemed to remove the film down my throat.

CREATING MY DAILY REPORT

Dealing with My Anger and Resentment

I was carrying a lot of anger and resentment about how and why I got injured and the lack of care and concern thereafter. Add to this litigation, WorkCover and over one hundred and eighty doctor's appointments at various locations, increased my breathing problems and my anxiety. I felt my emotions escalating trying to manage all the medical reports, juggling bills, finances, appointments and so forth and it was overwhelming. My past happy, passionate and positive disposition morphed into a frightened, angry and resentful demeanor.

My solution to these difficulties; I came to the conclusion that I was wasting my energy and time on thoughts about those who clearly had no care about my situation. I couldn't change the past but I could change how I used my energy and time and decided to redirect it into something useful to help me! I used it to focus on creating a management plan and system so I didn't feel so overwhelmed. Pulling myself out of the angry mode was challenging however my need to get things in order for the battle ahead was greater. I spoke with my psychologist and aired my feelings of anger and resentment and that made me feel better having someone to talk to and I needed to be productive as I had important work to do.

So, I pulled up my socks and mentally hired myself as my own "Personal Assistant". I had to stay clear-headed and get paperwork in order, so I was fully prepared for the barrage of reports needed in preparing myself for my extremely important legal case. I felt like I was going into battle and this needed my full attention and energy. I created a system to track and log outcomes from my breathing issues, meetings and medications etc. which proved valuable information for me, my doctors and lawyers.

I purchased some ring binders to sort my physical paperwork out and put companies, doctor's invoices, bills relating to my injury etc. into A – Z and within that, date order, so paperwork was easy for me to access. I also created spreadsheets on my computer (textbooks could be used to do the same thing) and had the following sheets/tabs/headings:-

Daily Report

- ➢ **Breathing issues** - date, time of issues, where I was, why it happened, trigger (if known), rating of breathing issue 1 – 5 (1 minor – 5 extremely severe)
- ➢ **Medication** – what is it, strength, prescribed by who, date taken, time taken, how I feel during and after taking it.
- ➢ **Appointments** - date, time, who, why, where, outcome (this had more detail)
- ➢ **Doctors** - name, address, phone number, date seen, outcome (this was in brief)

- ➤ **Lawyers** - name, address, phone number, date seen, outcome (this was in brief)
- ➤ **Workcover** - name, address, phone number, date seen, outcome (this was in brief)
- ➤ **Employer** - name, address, phone number, date seen, outcome (this was in brief)

**It was very important that I filled in my Daily Report
at the end of <u>EVERY DAY</u>.**

I also created a new contact in my mobile phone called "A Daily Update" and put in MY phone number. This enabled me to write an immediate SMS message to myself explaining quick details about a breathing issue or appointments etc. that I could read later and elaborate on when I was typing or writing in my Daily Report.

Being able to empty this information out of my head each night and place it into my Daily Report where it was organized, detailed and easy to access was extremely important, useful and reduced my stress.

Even if you're not going through litigation and newly learning about your triggers, I believe it could still be a helpful tool.

Why not create below what your Daily Report would look like?
What headings would you have?
What information would be useful to you?

Dealing with my Drama, Fear, Panic, Anxiety and Stress

The drama, fear, panic, anxiety and stress I felt depleted my energy and brain power and plagued me during or after each onslaught of breathing issues, which were unpredictable and at times extremely frightening. I was isolated and on a first name basis with the paramedics whom I'd never had to call in my life prior to this injury.

I began to recognize conversations that highlighted the same victim mentality loop I had been in, pre-empting disaster even before getting off the sofa and I was in a fearful and stressed survival holding pattern with no runway to land on and no-where to offload these draining emotions. It left me feeling powerless and that was awful.

Having respiratory difficulties is part of my life with RADS however that didn't mean I couldn't reduce my triggers or have a goal to eliminate them. I no longer wanted to live like a scared kitten and have a "victim" mentality. It was **time to step up** and create solutions to change this part of my life.

I had to be **ready and willing** to accept change, not only physical, also **how** and **what** I **thought** and what I **told myself** was **extremely important**.

I was sick of being sick and it was time, it was **MY TIME** to invest my good energy into changing these parts of my life and my routine. **I made a choice** to fight like a Warrior and no longer live in fear and **only I could do that!**

(Even if you don't initially embrace a strong Can-Do mindset, yet you still practice these strategies, then the good news is, don't be surprised if their success sneaks up on you. Making the effort to practice as often as you can is very important.)

My solution to these difficulties; Being committed and embracing a **Can-Do** mindset, putting in the time and energy and working on me because **I REALLY** wanted **better for myself**. I knew for significant change to happen; I had to **REALLY WANT IT** and **BELIEVE** it **COULD** and **WOULD** happen!

When I was having breathing issues, drama, fear, panic, stress and anxiety were draining my good energy and prolonging the situation, so **I HAD ENOUGH** and decided, they were **NO LONGER INVITED!**

I repeat, they were <u>NO LONGER INVITED</u>!

I created the visualization below to make positive and necessary changes and I practiced it repeatedly for success.

If you use your imagination and try to see the scenario below like a short movie in your mind. I would practice this in a quiet and peaceful setting when my mind was still.

Also, try not to judge or over analyze it, instead focus on the images and what is happening in the story in your mind and <u>what you want to achieve</u>. Put aside that it may all sound a little odd or silly because I am living proof it can work!

Don't underestimate the power of your mind!

You could use my visualization, modify it or create your own or work with a mental health professional to assist you in creating one specific to your needs. If it helps you during and/or after a breathing issue, that's wonderful!

I made my visual larger than life, colorful and very animated, and decided on a male genie, however your genie could be female or an animal or whatever you like, so here we go: -

"I imagine I have my own personal big genie with massive arms crossed standing at huge wooden doors that have **MY NAME** engraved on them. The genie's job is to guard those doors because behind them, my life is in progress. The genie looks down at these sniveling little trolls creeping up to the door and they are called drama, fear, panic, anxiety and stress who are trying to get in and attach to me each time I have a breathing issue. So, the genie glares down at them saying, **"YOU ARE NOT ON THE LIST, (insert your name) HAS IMPORTANT WORK TO DO AND NEEDS ALL THEIR ENERGY, SO LEAVE NOW!"** With that, the genie stomps their foot and the whole ground shakes and presto, those draining little trolls all turn and run off and dissolve as they run!"

As an add on … as I come out the door to thank my genie he gives me a massive hug and I feel safe and really proud that we worked as a team!

(If a hug isn't your thing then he/she could give you a "high five" instead. Whatever works for you to feel good about your accomplishment.)

With that, I was free and it felt **SO GOOD** because I had made the choice to **NEVER** allow those emotions to attach or invade my headspace when I had a breathing issue. I had serious work to do with my RADS and I couldn't effectively accomplish following my Plan of Action with them draining and distracting me, so I had to put my foot down (via my genie).

The choice WAS mine and I was the ONLY person who had the POWER to change it…so I DID!

Although this happened quite fast for me, I kept practicing it over and over to ensure **I was now in control**.

A few other suggestions could be to have the words drama, fear, panic, anxiety and stress simply fly off on a cloud into the air or the genie could simply blow the words away, or you could replace the genie with a Drill Sergeant. You can be as animated and colorful as you like, as long as it's effective and works when you need it most.

The result I wanted was **ME taking back control of ME** in times when I need to get on with an important job and it **WORKED** and has worked every single time since. How very cool is that!

To practice, you could also try role-playing whatever scenario you use and keep practicing it over and over, so when you do need it to happen in a "real situation," it does smoothly and without effort.

Over time and with practice it freed up my headspace and energy and I felt calmer and in control and was able to swiftly move forward with my Plan of Action when a breathing issue presented.

An important note, I only avert these particular emotions during or after a breathing issue to enable me to calmly implement my strategies. I recognize in different situations some of these emotions may be useful and important.

It's also a good idea to discuss different strategies with your mental health professional and together you could work on one that suits your specific needs.

You could use the page below to write down words or a scene that you would find helpful.

I created the idiom "Air Detective" because with my new heightened sense of smell that was the new Super Power I had been gifted. I was now using it constantly assessing every molecule of air I breathed and that became draining and exhausting. My challenge was to harness these amazing powers and figure out how to get the "assessing of air" part under control as I knew it would assist my physical and mental health.

The fact I could now smell a multitude of scents, toxins, smoke at one hundred paces was quite incredible to me and I would often jokingly say I could be hired out as a walking air quality control officer.

I had already created my Plan of Action (below) and that was important because my Chief Air Assessor had to direct me to it.

Learning how to be an efficient Air Detective and reducing stress and fear took time to develop because I was initially hypervigilant. I had to streamline and delegate the work of assessing the air, so I didn't get so worn out and frazzled because it was a 24 hour job, 7 days a week.

I closed my eyes and with the use of visualization and some creative elements, I designed, in my mind, a friendly character with a very special huge nose that had amazing smelling abilities. He was now my "Chief Air Assessor" and I made it his fulltime job to sniff and assess the air I breathe. He's a wonderful character who never gets flustered, never takes a day off and never asks for a pay rise!

Below is my rough drawing of my Chief Air Assessor .. You get the picture.. I know, I can't draw but I gave it a shot.

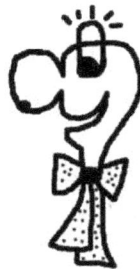

In the past I would feel fear and panic with red flags waving madly in my mind when there was compromised air however after implementing my friendly Chief Air Assessor, he would give me his valued opinion about the air so there was no need for stress, panic or fear. In a very calm and matter of fact way, he would deliver his verdict of the air quality and after much practice, this all happens in seconds.

I share the following visual with you: -

In the back blocks of my mind, I would imagine him laying back in an old non-smelling recliner sofa just quietly assessing the air quality every single second of every day and only when needed would he pop into my thoughts with a knowing warm look on his face and calmly say, "the airs not great right now, time to start one of your Plans of Action".

Within a flash the appropriate Plan of Action springs to mind and I do it, without any red flags or stress, **I just get on with it**.

In those few seconds he (I) have: -

ASSESSED the air quality and based on how strong the smell is etc. I will then…
ACT on it by implementing one of my Plans of Action as I am moving away from it, and once I am safe and my breathing is getting under control, I will then...
ANALYISE what the smell was, where it came from and determine how I can avoid, reduce or eliminate it.

To become an Air Detective takes practice and you too can create your own friendly little Chief Air Assessor character (or pop up message or whatever works for you) in your mind, just remember to make it "drama-free" and as colorful or as animated as you like. Once you put your character to work keeping a nose on the air quality, you can move forward with the best Plan of Action for that situation.

I also feel having Air Detective skills is great for the whole family to try as I've spoken to some people with RADS who have supportive partners and loved ones and it's heart-warming to hear how they also turn into Air Detectives. Some will assess a room before they allow their partner to go in or help to check the air quality when they are out and about.

Becoming an Air Detective and passing that job over to my Chief Air Assessor has been an important tool in enabling me to reduce my triggers and mange my breathing issues in a calm and sensible way.

Tip…A RADS Warrior friend recently reminded me of all the great apps now available that can also help us check air quality in various locations, wind, temperature, emergency services etc.

Why not draw below what your Chief Air Assessor would look like and what name you would give them? It would be great to hear from you with a picture of your creation.

CREATING A "PLAN OF ACTION"

These days, if I come into contact with a trigger, combining my Air Detective skills, my Genie and my Plan of Action means I now have the tools to assist in the management of my breathing issues and I am able to leave my home more often. **How GREAT is that!**

Prior to developing the above tools, after I was diagnosed with RADS and I was home, I put in place the steps below to help reduce my fear and stress. Now I have moved to a different location and home, I rarely need to implement this, which I am very happy about, however, I share it with you in the hope you may find it useful.

In the first year after my injury and I was home, I was experiencing a multitude of breathing issues every day because I was yet to understand what and how to identify a trigger and reduce or remove them. Below is what I would do to get through this very difficult time.

*** MY INSIDE "PLAN OF ACTION" ***

First is preparation and this comprised of the following;

I chose a particular song on my phone that I found relaxing and calming and I called that my **RADS calming song**. I _only_ play it during or after an exposure. This is _**very**_ important! I made a collage from photos of the beach, showing people breathing well and I put them all on one piece of paper, printed it out and put it on the front of my fridge. I wrote out in BIG print a list of six instructions **TO DO** if I was having a breathing issue at home and stuck that list on my fridge door.

Some breathing issues were quite severe and I found it hard to talk or think constructively, so having guidelines written out in **BIG** print (so I didn't need to find my glasses to read it) was very helpful. I knew to go straight to the kitchen, look at the fridge and start reading and follow my instructions: -

1/ Turn on the extraction fan above the stove – as the movement of air helped to settle my airways. (I did this prior to owning an air purifier or having my medical air and oxygen tanks)

2/ Turn on your RADS calming song and slow down

3/ Make a warm drink or use the steam cup to settle your airways

4/ Look at the picture on the fridge of the beach and people breathing clean air and calm down

5/ Use positive internal language to calm yourself

**S L O W EVERYTHING DOWN**
**I AM GOING TO GET THROUGH THIS**
**S L O W YOUR BREATHING DOWN**
**YOU ARE DOING SO WELL!** _Repeat_

6/ If you are having any difficulties through these steps or not managing then call 000 or Emergency

(Obviously change number 6/ with your countries emergency number.)

Once my breathing had settled and due to the fact my breathing issues are always from a trigger, I would try to identify the trigger and do what I could do to rectify, remove or change the situation in an effort to prevent it happening again.

Having my **TO DO** list above, helped to reduce my fear and stress and I felt like a well-trained soldier following my plan and for me, it worked!

You can create your own Inside "Plan of Action" or modify mine or speak to your health professional and create strategies that suit your particular needs.

This taught me I also needed an Outside "Plan of Action" so I worked on directives and different techniques to manage the breathing issues I experienced outside my home.

Now having invented my Chief Air Assessor, who's working quietly in the back blocks of my mind, he has become extremely good at being able to assess the air quality very fast and then I can determine the level of urgency for each exposure and go straight to my Plan of Action.

The fact I practiced this over and over means I now do it without even thinking as it's become second nature, like riding a bike. I just get on with whatever needs to be done and do it.

Drama, fear, panic, stress and anxiety are not invited and my Genie ensures they are kept away at these times because I have important work to do and I need to focus.

Below are some typical scenarios:-

Scenario 1
I can smell something (not overly strong) that is causing my airway to have a slight reaction. It might have been the end of day aftershave someone is wearing or I have walked toward a new timber fence that is off-gassing.
Scenario 2
I can smell or taste the trigger and it's quite strong and I can feel a reaction happening i.e. I start to clear my throat and cough, my voice may go croaky and I start to experience breathing difficulties. It might have been from someone walking past me with newly applied perfume or I walk past someone smoking and wasn't quick enough to hold my breath.
Scenario 3
I can immediately smell or taste a very strong trigger and my airways become very reactive and I have immediate breathing issues and I may also be coughing and I may not be able to speak. It could be from inhaling diesel fumes or the smell of newly laid bitumen.
Scenario 4
I cannot identify any particular smell or taste however I can feel my airways starting to react, I start to cough and my voice changes to a raspy sound. This may be from a chemical or toxin similar to what I experienced when

exposed to formaldehyde or when I tried a new no VOC paint. (it is important to know that not all triggers have smells, so feel and listen to your body)

<u>Regardless of which scenario,</u>
<u>if I have any breathing issues</u>
<u>I follow my Plan of Action below:-</u>

*** MY OUTSIDE "PLAN OF ACTION" ***

❖ **Get myself AWAY from the trigger**

❖ **Go to a safe clean air environment**
- I might get into my vehicle and turn on the air-conditioning
- Go home and turn on my air purifier or prior to having that, I would put the extraction fan on above my stove and allow the moving air to help settle my airways
- Go to the beach, if it's a good air day with wind blowing in the right direction and sit or lay down in or out of my vehicle
- Go to the forest and sit down at a good air spot or sit or lay in my vehicle with the window down
- Go into a large shop that I know has very good air-conditioning and sit down
- At any time if needed, call 000 *(or your countries emergency number)* or go to hospital

I would then either simultaneously or immediately after implementing one of the above, do some or all of the strategies below to best help me at that time: -

❖ Use my medical air or oxygen
❖ Put on my charcoal activated mask
❖ Gargle clean water and spit out contents and do this a few times
❖ Use my positive internal language to remain calm, focused and encourage and praise myself on doing well
❖ Use my positive internal language to remind myself to slow down my breathing.
❖ Use my hand-held fan to slowly fluff clean air toward me
❖ Chew gum to create saliva down my throat and help to keep my throat saturated
❖ Use my steam cup to gently fluff warm steam toward me
❖ Play my RADS calming song
❖ Assess my breathing and if I need assistance or was not managing

then call Emergency 000 (or your countries emergency number) or go to hospital

Once my breathing issue subsided and I was in a safe air environment I would then:-

❖ Analyze what the trigger was (if known), where it came from and determine how I can avoid, reduce or eliminate it in the future and store that useful information in my mind.

****

I am usually highly reactive after a strong trigger, so I would isolate myself until my airways have settled. Lying down is very effective in helping me to recover and I may also play my RADS calming music or meditate, which is extremely helpful.

I have been caught in my van when there was a major fire ahead and I could not turn around and had to drive through thick smoke for what felt like ages but it was probably a couple of minutes. I started my Plan of Action the moment I saw and smelt the smoke and began working through what I needed to do. I put on my mask (with the charcoal activated filter) and closed all my windows tight. I turned off my van's air-conditioning, grabbed a hand towel and dampened it with some water from my water bottle and draped it over my mask without covering the outlet valve. I turned my tank of medical air on low and fed the tube under my mask near my mouth and started giving myself a positive pep talk. I was now prepared and ready to drive through the smoke ahead. Sadly, there was nowhere to turn around and it was a one-way road, so I just had to follow the traffic in front of me. I could feel my adrenalin rising as I was driving through the thickest of smoke however my positive self-talk kept me in check and although a hint of the smell of smoke came into my van, doing the above did a good enough job to give me time to get out of the area. I felt like I was running a military-type operation and it ran smoothly with a successful outcome. Eventually, I was able to air out my van, my masks and felt relieved and very proud of a job well done!

I have also been driving out on a highway and when I looked in my mirror, I saw a massive dust storm chasing me. So, I went straight into my Plan of Action and safely and quickly pulled off the road, closed all my air vents and windows, turned off my air-conditioning and just for some added protection I put a small dust mask inside my heavy-duty charcoal filtered mask. I turned on my tank of medical air and put the tube under the chin of my masks. I had my water bottle and empty bottle close and then I looked up on my phone where the closest hospital was in the event I needed to head there. I put on my hazard lights and saw the massive rolling cloud of dust about to engulf my van. Although it was an intense situation, I had practiced and used my Plan of Action so many times I just went into autopilot and did everything I needed to do to be safe. While I could feel adrenalin pumping, I made an effort to slow my breathing down so I could concentrate on assessing the air without drama or panic distracting me. *(Below you can see the dust storm in my revision mirror. It was massive!)*

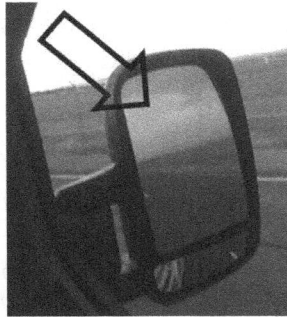

Below is a recollection of the self-talk I did:-

"You are doing such a good job... before you know it you will be off driving again... Nice slow breaths ... that's good... breathe in two three four .. breathe out two three four.. How lovely and clean is the air being pumped into your masks right now... it feels good doesn't it... You have heaps of medical air in the tank so you're going to be fine... It's getting closer .. you'll be ok ... I wonder if the next town has a place to wash my van... You're doing really well.... It's going to pass soon and you'll be on the other side of it.... Oh here it comes....wow it's windy and rocking the van .... how good is this clean air you're breathing in right now and having two masks is helping because no taste of dust...I wonder how animals cope with this.... poor things....who would have thought that dust could be so red in colour. Oh it's all dark now... I must be in the middle of it... hmm interesting... my masks are working well...I feel like I'm in a dirty cloud and still my air feels good and I can't smell any dust... so that's good... Oh the rocking is easing... there's some light coming through so it's going to be over soon. You're doing so great and your van is going to really need a good wash.... Nice slow breaths.. in two three four.. slowly .. out two three four...you're doing really well... it's nearly over and look at that you're coming out the other side... Your Plan of Action worked really well....well done, you did a GREAT job!"

I remember getting out of my van after it passed and just standing on the side of the road feeling quite emotional while I watched the dust storm roll off into the distance. I was thinking how very glad I was to have my Plan of Action and medical air and to not have ended up in hospital!

Utilizing the strategies and my Plan of Action, prepares me for any situation and has enabled me to manage and cope more confidently with different triggers. No longer having drama to disrupt and drain me, I can get on with what I need to do and this has been an enormous and significant part of my success. Sometimes I will improvise and use things like other masks or the towel etc. Just whatever I feel I need to help me remain safe and get through a situation.

Now that you have read what I do, you could design your own Plan of Action or modify mine or work with your medical professional to create one that works specifically for you.

Remember, if ever you have a breathing issue and need assistance and you weren't managing then call Emergency 000 (or whatever number in your country) or go to hospital.

TIP... In case of an extreme Emergency and if I've run out of medical air or oxygen and can't speak, I have a written note in my phone cover that explains I have RADS and not asthma and inhalers don't work for me, I just need clean air, medical air or oxygen and here is my doctor and specialist's number. This could be given to paramedics or medical staff. To date I've not needed to use it as I make sure I always have a spare full tank of oxygen in the back of my van.

Once you know what helps you, you could use the space below to start creating your Plan of Action for inside your home and one for outside.
It would be great to hear what solutions and strategies you use or create.

THERAPIES AND SELF HELP

Joy, Laughter and Music

Now having RADS, I felt my life had turned grey and gloomy and it became a struggle to find any joy because I had to avoid outside activities and isolate myself for too long.

Once I had my tools and Plan of Action in place, I decided to do something about this side of my life because joy laughter and music is essential for our health and wellbeing. So, I started to watch funny videos on the internet that made me laugh, as well as pictures that made me feel good. Dog videos, cat videos, music videos, babies laughing videos, proposal videos and on and on, I had an endless supply! I made a habit of watching some before I went to bed, so my mind was full of sweet happy thoughts and then I could calmly chill out and do my end of night visualization and meditation.

If I was feeling down or lonely, I would make an effort to wear my most colorful shirt or dress and play some of my favorite music and that made me feel good, light and vibrant.

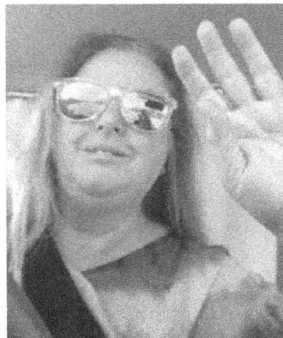

Sure, it was a distraction but it was a **good** distraction and sometimes when I felt good, I would sing or dance around my living room like no-one was watching … because no-one was! I made an effort to turn on the music a few times a week and I know it helped me. I also started to play music in my van and sing when I went out or if I was away travelling. You've never heard anyone belt out "Baby Did A Bad Bad Thing" while crossing the Nullarbor alone in a van like I did. I'm sure the kangaroos and lizards loved it!

When's the last time you turned up the radio when a cool song was playing and sang along?

At times it was hard work finding joy but the more I practiced every day I was surprised how empowering it was and motived me to continue because I knew what I was teaching myself was working. It was good to inject some happiness into my world and smile again.

Speaking of smiling, don't underestimate how much positive impact the act of smiling can have on your health! Just check the internet and read what the experts say about smiling and you might be surprised! So, I make an effort to watch a good comedy or read good jokes and have a laugh because I am now aware what an important tool it is and I try to do it as often as I can! In fact, I'm doing it right now!

Meditation

I have found meditation to be wonderful in assisting me to relax and have used it in many aspects of my life. It's also been very beneficial for aiding my recovery from a trigger. In my case, I need to lay-down to have the most effective recovery from sore lungs and I used to get impatient and bored. Once I started to use different relaxation and breathing techniques to slip into a beautiful meditation it helped me to release impatience and allow my body to heal.

I am aware there are hundreds if not thousands of meditations on the internet, so you have a huge choice.

At night before I go to sleep, I practice meditating after I have done my visualization. This allows my mind to settle and drift into a peaceful sleep and below I share a little about what I do.

I start by laying down and relaxing my head, neck and shoulders to lay gently and ease into my pillow. I breathe in slowly and imagine my lungs filling up with lovely clean air and think about the last time I walked at the beach with my puppy and I begin to smile as I slowly breathe out. I think about how nice it is to just relax and take another slow breath in and allow my hands to just fall open and relax as I slowly breathe out and smile again. I slowly relax each part of my body, my arms, my fingers, chest, lungs and concentrate on each body part, taking slow breaths in and slow breaths out, allowing my belly to rise and fall gently. I say thank you in my mind to my body for doing such a wonderful job and working so well.

You could also listen to music or enjoy the silence and think of nothing. Whatever works for you and helps you to feel calm and relaxed.

Positive Affirmations

I have little messages around my home like "**Today is a GOOD day!**" and "**Wish it Dream it DO IT**" and I also write uplifting notes on my message board like "**Create, Design, Accomplish!**" and "**You Can Do It!**" All are encouraging reminders that help motivate me and maintain a healthy and positive mindset.

Positive Self Talk, the Language I Use

I do Positive Self Talk a lot! Mostly saying **I CAN** and **I AM**. I usually repeat a particular important message I feel I need to hear twenty to hundreds of times in my head. I might say, "**I AM going to be OK today when I go out,**" or "**You have your PLAN, so you CAN handle anything**!" and so forth. I believe this is also a great jumpstart in helping me reboot and maintaining a positive mindset.

If things don't go as well as expected, then I don't stress but rather think about what I can learn from the experience and what I would change for next time, file it away under useful information and not dwell on it. It's that simple!

I believe words you say to yourself or even the dialogue in conversations you have with others is also important and since it was pointed out to me, I make a big effort to focus on positives. Previously, I could hear myself being negative, overly dramatic and inciting doom saying comments like; "I'm NEVER going to do x or y again, or I'm TERRIFIED to step out my front door, or EVERY TIME I go out, I have triggers, or my triggers can be so bad I CAN'T do anything!" etc.

This was the kind of language I used and it would spin around in my head keeping me in a constant state of fear and misery.

Once I changed my words to; "**Although it might be challenging, I AM going to find a way to do x and y**" or "**Today will be a GOOD day and if I have a trigger, I AM prepared because I have a plan!** "

Once I had practiced over and over using my new tools and my Plan of Action to manage my triggers, I felt confident and empowered and I changed my dialogue and self-chatter and my world started to look a whole lot better.

I understand we can all have bad days and bad weeks but when it turns into bad months, I believe it can become our language, so it's good to be made aware of it because like me, you might not even know you're doing it. Try listening to the words you use and how you say them as they leave your mouth and you may be surprised!

Choose to want better for yourself, I would repeat this mantra every day, twice a day;

**I DESERVE BETTER AND THE CHANGES I MAKE,
EVEN SMALL ONES ARE GOOD!
I KNOW I CAN DO IT!
I WANT TO DO IT!
IT'S TIME.. IT'S MY TIME !
I AM READY!**

Repeat

Now being sensible here, I didn't go running off out the front door and nor should you!

Being motived to change meant I was on my way and that's very exciting but there was still more work to do in practicing to use the tools to help with my breathing issues.

Something that happened soon after I made a number of changes, I will share with you.

I used to say "I won't EVER be able to go to the little dance club because everyone wears perfume and it's just TOO HARD", so I changed it to "I love to go to the little dance club to listen to the music and see people enjoy themselves, so I WILL find some way to do it." and I became proactive and positive and I really meant what I said and I believed it could happen and once I had the tools to manage my breathing issues.. guess what, it DID HAPPEN! I didn't stay for too long but I had a couple of dances and for the time I was there, I had a great time and just knowing I accomplished it, made me feel **very** good!

Once I started my positive dialogue, I began adding more mantras and I would say them with determination, passion and excitement.

"I **AM** going to cope in a much calmer way when I have a breathing issue, I **AM** committed to making the changes I need and I know **I CAN** do it! I am **READY** to do the work!"

I would say that over and over and with it came feelings of excitement.

You can use the same mantra's I use, modify them or create new positive ones yourself. Sometimes I would say some of mine out loud when I'm driving my van or when I'm laying down at the end of a day. No matter where, when or how I say them, I make sure I do and I believe what I say to myself!

For some folks, this might all sound a little "out there" however, why not give it a try? Better that you think and talk about positive things in your mind or out loud rather than flood your mind and energy with negative or sad thoughts.

Don't underestimate the power of your mind!
You have the CHOICE about what you want to think!

(Just think about that for a moment and read it again and again)

****

Important Reminder:- please reach out and speak to your doctor or mental health professional if you are not coping or need assistance with your mental health.

If you have a favorite and uplifting mantra, why not send me an email to share yours, as it would be nice to read what is positive and helpful to you.

Self-Check

One night I was sitting on my sofa and I looked at my hands and noticed they were clenched and that my body felt tense. I took the steps of slowly breathing in and slowly breathing out and allowing my shoulders to sag down. I did it again and allowed my arms to go limp and repeated it, to allow my hands to rest and my body to relax. I just sat for a few moments to enjoy feeling like I had let out the air in a tyre that was pumped up a bit too much and was grateful I noticed it. I call this a "self-check" and made an effort to stop and "feel" how my body "feels" more often and repeated the above steps as needed.

Self-Hypnosis

Being a Practitioner of Hypnosis, I utilize these tools together with visualization and positive self-talk to help me remain focused during a trigger and I have also used it to invent creative and practical solutions. It has been an important component in assisting me to maintain a positive mindset and focus on good results and to influence my body to heal.

I recently used Self-Hypnosis, visualization and positive self-talk while in hospital having an operation without general anesthesia due to my RADS and it all went well. I also believe using these practices assisted my body to heal during recovery.

There are courses and books available about hypnosis and self-hypnosis and I list those that have been helpful to me in the back of my book.

Sleep, Diet and Exercise

Having good sleep sounds simple however having extremely sensitive airways I found that difficult to achieve due to the triggers I was having through the night waking me up or not allowing me to get to sleep. Once I was able to identify the triggers and remove them or myself from the situation, I was usually able to get sleep but this took some time to achieve, so I was initially very sleep deprived and my coping skills were frayed.

It is extremely important to get all the sleep you need so you can heal as without it, I noticed my healing process was prolonged. Using my tools such as meditation and self-talk assisted me and although I used to feel guilty sleeping nine or ten hours, in the end, I just decided that my body must need that time to repair.

Eating nutritional food and having a balanced diet is also really important. For me, my focus was so much on my breathing I developed poor eating habits. I began comfort eating and not exercising and this meant I put on a lot of weight. Over time I changed my diet and now try to focus on eating clean simple food like fish and steamed vegetables and I try to eat more fruit.

In regard to exercise, my respiratory sensitivities made going to the gym's I walked into impossible (see under Gyms), which escalated my frustration and coping ability, so I needed the support of my psychologist. Being an independent person made it difficult to ask for help and I needed to work on this.

My solution was I created a gym in my garage and I go through stages of motivation using the equipment and then if I have an exposure to something and I'm left with sore lungs, my gym workout falls away. Once I start missing a few days, that can turn into weeks however I do try to start using it again when I am well enough. At one stage in my previous home I wanted a safe place to walk/ exercise so I invested in a treadmill and that worked great, when I used it!

Now living close to the ocean, on good air days I can get out for nice little walks next to the beach and in 2019 I bought my puppy. So, she is great to walk with and she provides me with lots of love, joy and laughter and she's an excellent motivator as well.

I feel the breathing exercises I do when I am at the beach on good air days are extremely beneficial to my lung health. When I am at the ocean and if it's a good air day, I will make an effort to put in the time to do some simple concentrated breathing exercises. I will find a nice quiet spot to sit and allow my body to relax. Then I will breathe in through my nose, a long slow inhalation of lovely clean sea air and I can feel my lungs open up as I do this. Then I exhale through my mouth and slowly blow the air out, as if I am blowing through a straw and allow my shoulders and arms to relax. I will do this a number of times and then after just relax and enjoy the smell of the ocean and if the sun is out, I might catch a few safe rays of sunshine to help maintain my levels of Vitamin D, as I am aware how important that is too.

I have seen there are heaps of different breathing techniques on the internet as well as many gentle yoga moves. I have been known to put a mattress on the floor in my lounge room and do what is probably regarded as a bit of gentle stretching now and then. I feel it all goes to helping my general health.

Socializing and Joining Groups

With RADS came avoidance, isolation and more time at home. When I was well enough to go out, my most social outing was going to the supermarket. Making it to the doors could be a challenge due to the fumes from cars and as long as I kept away from the strong-smelling isles and people with scented products, I would do well. The staff knew me and as sad as this is to admit, those lovely staff behind the counter in the deli (where it was always nice and cold with good air) would be my source of human contact and conversation for many months.

Friendships are important to foster and maintain and socializing was something I had to work on and feeling confident to successfully get out more was a three-year process due to developing the tools I needed and learning what appropriate strategy to implement to be safe. This all took a lot of practice over those years.

The night before I was planning to go out, I would visualize myself walking, smiling, feeling good and see myself in whatever situation I was planning on doing. Before walking out the door I would look in the mirror and say to myself "You've got this! You know what to do if you come into contact with a trigger, so relax and enjoy yourself!" I might be going for a walk, heading off to the library or post office. If things didn't go as well as I had visualized, I thought about what I could do different and learn from it and over time I had stored helpful information in my mind to draw on if and when needed, without drama or panic.

Eventually I felt more comfortable going out and I met a wonderful couple who never wear any scented products and are terrific company and are now close friends. I also make an effort to go and visit my family and friends who now know and understand my sensitivities and are very considerate not to wear products that trigger me. I consider myself very fortunate and also try to go out to lunch or dinner at least once a month and I can't tell you how great it is! Although I can't predict who's going to turn up wearing something that might cause me to have a reaction, I now have my tools and Plan of Action and I am sensible where I sit (see under Restaurants) and what to do if I come into contact with a trigger.

So more often than not, I get to stay with and enjoy my friends, food and great conversation and that's wonderful!

The RADS International Facebook Group is also great to pop in and have a chat with other people with RADS. My intention when I first set up the group was to unite people with RADS and I'm really proud it's happening by way of this group and it's a good forum to chat about all the challenges we face living with such a unique condition.

Closer to home, I am aware shires and councils can also offer different support groups and activities you may find interesting.

Having my campervan, I wanted to travel but I didn't want to head off on my own and would have loved to have another traveler convoy with me, so I joined an online travel group for people who went away traveling in their motorhomes and caravans etc. Initially I had a lot of people interested in wanting to convoy with me and I have to say I was very excited as I had spent so much time on my own. Sadly, once it got close to making a time to leave, people started to cancel and, in the end, no-one would travel with me. I was confused and upset and later someone confided in me, that it was due to my sensitivities of not being able to be near cigarette smoke, campfires or scented products.

I felt utterly miserable and took a few days out feeling sorry for myself, then I pulled up my socks and thought "stuff that, get over it" and decided fear wasn't going to stop me and if no-one would travel with me then I would do a trip on my own!

I decided to make a **RADS Awareness Trip across Australia.**

The fact I was initially misdiagnosed by so many doctors, I decided I would drop off flyers about RADS and the support I was offering for those newly diagnosed. In total, I called into 36 hospital as well as many doctors' rooms and hand-delivered thousands of flyers. Every person I spoke to had never heard of RADS, so I felt it was really worthwhile. I also took videos along the way so I didn't feel so alone and to document my journey.

I drove from Melbourne Victoria, Australia all the way over to the other side of Australia to Perth Western Australia and then I drove all the way back, which was thousands of kilometers. I tried to drive near the coast as much as I could as my airways always felt better near the ocean and I saw some amazing sights. I posted my little movie on YouTube "RADS Awareness Trip across Australia Part 1 and Part 2" and hoped other people with RADS might see it and be inspired. I have to say I was really proud to have accomplished that trip, especially on my own.

(Below I stopped and took a shot of the very long road across the Nullabor)

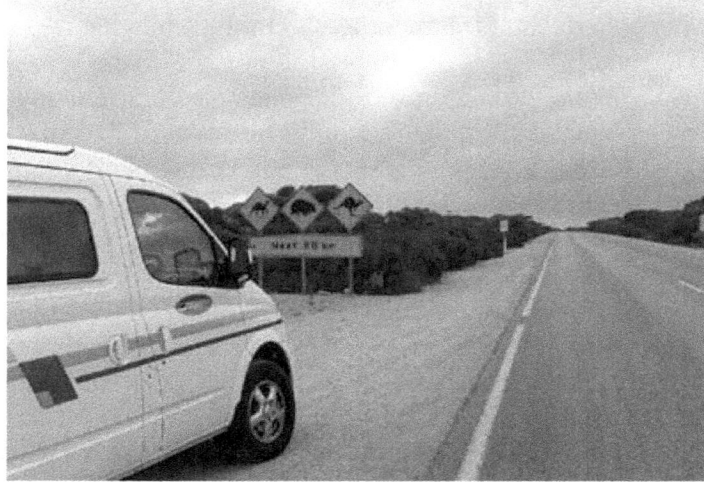

Using my Plan of Action and other strategies to remain calm along the way when faced with difficult air situations and having everything in the van from my RADS Tool Kit, proved successful and was a great learning experience. It boosted my confidence that although I would have preferred to travel in convoy with another van, I could travel and do things on my own even having RADS.

While joining groups would be great from a social aspect, I can't control who is going to turn up wearing something that may cause me breathing issues however I won't let that dampen my enthusiasm because maybe no-one will turn up wearing any fragrance! I will continue and keep trying and feel sure sometime in the future I will get lucky and find a fun social group I can attend and not get triggered and we chat about light and fun things.

In the meantime, maybe a social "Scent Free Group" to go to dinner or the movies etc. would be something I need to think about creating sometime?

It's no fun feeling lonely and the only way to change that is to do something about it.

Why not use the space below to write out three of your favorite songs, three movies you would like to watch, three places you would like to visit and your top three exercises? I know, I'm struggling to find one exercise, as sadly I don't think opening the fridge door counts as an exercise.

Visualization

Since I was young, having a vivid imagination was useful and I practiced visualization before I even knew the word, so although I have not had any formal training, I have been doing it for decades and used that and the skills I learnt in hypnosis to fine-tune my mental imagery.

I use visualization for many situations, like preparing myself for the following day or days when I know I have appointments where I may be exposed to triggers or events happening in my life or to forward plan happy, positive and successful outcomes. I have found it to be an extremely powerful and valuable asset in my creative toolbox and something I find simple to do. Like anything, if you practice it enough, it becomes easier to do. I know people who use visualization to find a good parking spot, which I do as well and why not!

Below is a visual I created that I sometimes use for slowing down the after-effects of a trigger.

If you think about what a field of wheat, high grass or bamboo moving gently in the breeze looks like, swaying slowly back and forth, that's how I imagine the tiny hairs (cilia) in my airway are like, just very tiny and swaying nice and calm. Then if I am exposed to a trigger, the wind has picked up and it's now blowing all the fine hairs in every direction. As I remove myself from the trigger and find clean air and implement one of my Plans of Action, I visualize the tiny hairs in my airway slowly and gently settling back to a gentle sway. Doing this along with positive self-talk has been very helpful.

DEVICES

Air Purifier

I have a lightweight triple hepa filter air purifier that has a timer and I can take it away with me. It is easy to clean the filter and it does a good job.

I also have a larger air purifier that has an "ionizer" button and when I turned it on, I could taste what I can only describe as a metal taste in the air and my breathing became labored. So I never have that button on.

My large heavy-duty air purifier and my smaller one had a good workout recently to keep smoke out of my safe room (my living room) in my new home during the massive bushfires here in Australia where smoke was carried for many kilometers through the air. They worked very well and kept my air smoke-free in my safe room.

It's important to do your own research about devices to suit your budget and needs. The internet is a great resource.

Humidifier

I have purchased two humidifiers and they both omit a very fine mist of cool steam into the air. I've not had any success with either helping my breathing issues and they have left my top blanket damp from the mist. It has been suggested to me to try using it at a different time of the year, so I might give one another try during summer and see how I go.

Oxygen Concentrator

When I first spoke about the prospect of trying an oxygen concentrator with my Respiratory Specialist, he pointed out a very important fact. He suggested they may not be able to provide 100% guarantee that the filter system would not be compromised if it was operating in a situation where there was smoke or fumes in the air. So, I did some research and contacted a few companies that sold them and none I found were able to provide the 100% guarantee I needed.

The fact I spend a fair amount of time in my van and I have been faced with smoke and fumes coming into the cabin of my van, I need 100% clean air to help me breathe and I can get this from my medical air tank. If you have found an oxygen concentrator that works for you, then that's great and it would be good to hear of your experience.

AIR IN A CAN

I discussed with my doctor, that I wanted to do a trial using a product that had "air in a can" and I was going to do my personal research first and be very cautious in doing my trial. I thought the product might come in handy to dissipate a small trigger, if I was just popping in and out of somewhere quick. Having my 5-kilo oxygen tank in my van gives me added peace of mind, however, I thought this was worth looking into because it's light and easy to carry and could be a second alternative, if it worked for me.

I learnt that canned air is also called "harvested" air and I asked a number of questions before testing the product. I wanted to know where their air came from and what kind of filtration system they had in place to filter the air they harvested. They also suggested other questions to ask, if I was approaching any other suppliers. Such as, are there any added chemicals, additives, supplements and other, is their air harvested overseas and if so where and does the product have anything in it that may affect a person's health. All important and good questions to ask!

I felt comfortable with the information they provided and that their product was of a very high standard, so I went forward with my trial.

Knowing how sensitive my airways are, I was extremely cautious when I first tried the air in a can. I held the can back about a foot from my mouth just to test the smell and taste of the air coming out. I wanted to test and see if I had any negative reaction when breathing it in and I didn't, so I moved the can a little closer and sprayed a little longer and still my airways were feeling good. Once I ascertained my airways were ok and I didn't have any negative reaction, I used it a number of times when I was out after having small exposures to scented products and it worked extremely well to dissipate the trigger. The can was about the same size as a large can of hairspray and it was very convenient to carry around as it fit in my large hand bag and was light as a feather.

Information to be mindful of from my personal use was, one can may only last about 130 inhalations, so when I used it for a continued spray of air for about 15 – 30 seconds it did a good job however not having an indicator of how much air is left in the can could place me in a dangerous situation if I need more clean air and couldn't get back to my van where my small oxygen tank is.

Maybe carrying two cans would be an option and taking into account where I am and how long I would be there etc. These are all variables I would need to think about if I was to use them again. The cans I had were a onetime use, so you cannot refill them and that can prove to be expensive for some of us.

For me, they were a convenient quick fix for short term use and handy to help dissipate small exposures if I was out.

Due to the fact our needs are all different with our RADS symptoms and some people have other health issues aside from RADS, it would be sensible to speak to your trusted health care professional before trying anything new and be guided by them, as well as doing your own research!

WALKING

Who would have thought that something as simple as just going for a walk could place me in a life-threatening situation? It's happened on several occasions and highlighted the importance of being extremely vigilant about air quality, wind and where and when I walk.

If people walk past me with certain perfume, aftershave, sun screen, insect repellents, lotions etc. it can cause me breathing issues that range from low to severe, depending on the intensity and concentration of the particular fume or smell.

Therefore, when I see people ahead and they are going to be walking past me, I usually move away to allow a large gap between us and I take in a slow breath of clean air before they walk past, then slowly let it out. Some can wear very strong fragrances that can linger and hang in the air for long distances, so I have learnt to take my time to exhale.

I am also very particular if I am walking anywhere there is traffic. I try to place myself so that any breeze is blowing fumes away from me and not toward me. Above all I try to avoid walking anywhere there is built up traffic and have favorite places that I have strategically checked for walking that are next to the ocean and away from traffic and well away from pollutants.

I recall a time I was walking along the beach on a gorgeous day but not too far from my van. Initially no-one else was around until one lady came jogging behind me and passed me and the breeze blew her strong perfume straight at me and I inhaled it. This all happened in seconds and it had me gasping for air, so I slowed everything down and gargled water from my bottle and slowly made my way back to my van. I laid down in my van and used some oxygen from my tank and eventually just allowed the sea air to do its job. It took a number of days for me to recover due to it being an extremely strong fragrance.

Now and then I might put my small oxygen tank in my backpack and head off on a bit longer walk if I have a friend with me. I'm sensible where I walk and ensure I have my phone charged and I have items with me from my RADS Tool Kit. If it's a bit dusty I might wear a mask or move to a different location. Fear no longer holds me back to get out and about because I'm sensible and have my management plan and tools ready if I am faced with breathing issues.

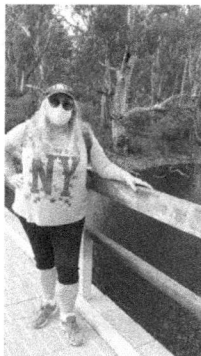

I also have some lovely little walking tracks very close to home and some big ovals to take my puppy and I usually head off with my water bottle in the middle of the day when no-one is around and zero traffic and as long it's not a northerly wind, we do pretty good.

I made a big decision to live near the ocean for my health. Moving wasn't easy to do however the outcome has provided me a better quality of life. Having good air quality that is trigger free is crucial in living the best life with RADS.

Prior to living near the ocean here at the Surf Coast, I would drive up to the forest instead as it was a lot closer to where I used to live and go for walks on tracks I knew to be safe for my breathing.

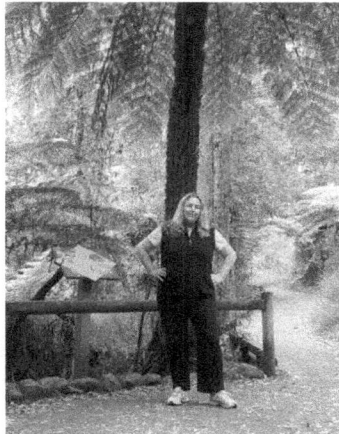

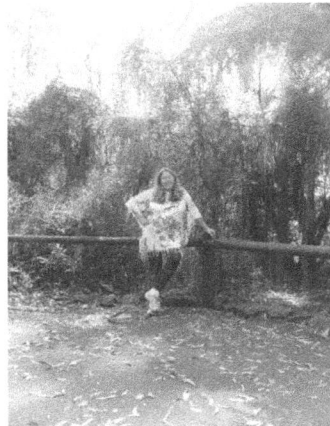

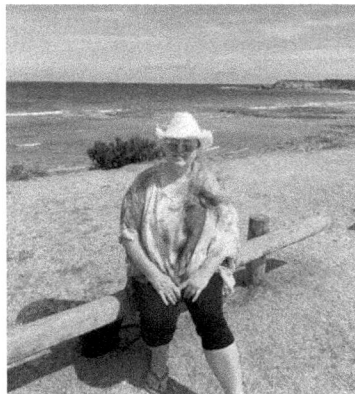

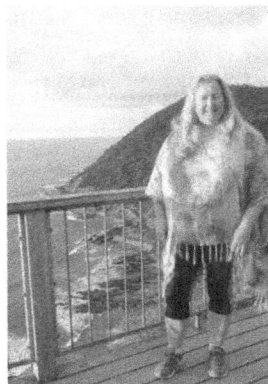

Checking the Air Quality

In the back-blocks of my mind, my Chief Air Assessor is lazing back rocking in his recliner chair constantly assessing the air with his big nose, so I don't need to think too much about it as he's doing his job. It just happens automatically now as he's been doing it for years and I know I can rely on him because he never takes a day off and has never let me down. All the practicing I did paid off!

I help out by trying to spend time at places that have the best air quality and for me, that's usually at the beach with the breeze blowing in with no pollutants.

I was recently visiting friends on the other side of town not far from a bay and I can't tell you how terrible the air quality was. All I could taste and smell were petrol fumes in the air and realized there was an oil refinery a few miles away and the wind was blowing the fumes across the bay.

On another occasion, I visited a person where their home was close to swamp land and the smell of stagnant water was extremely strong and caused me breathing issues. I've also visited someone near the beach on the other side of town and the smell of the seaweed was so strong we had to leave the beach.

When building my home in a new area I didn't consider how much the new building smells would impact the air quality. On days the wind blew in from the north I could smell epoxy, pine, and paint fumes which are all triggers for me, so I spent a lot of time in my van, away from the area.

If you are looking to re-locate or going away on holiday, then consider what is nearby to you that could impact on the air quality and your breathing. Also think about what time of year farmers might harvest or burn off etc.

Sadly, as I write this there are massive fires burning out of control across Australia devastating the land and people and animals are tragically losing their lives. The usual pristine beaches here along the coast are being enveloped in smoke blowing down from these fires and I am into my fourth day of what I call "lockdown" to keep safe. Please check under Smoke – for more details in regard to how and what I do.

There are now helpful apps and websites to provide information about air quality around the world, so if you do a search on the internet you should find some. There are also some mentioned in our Facebook Group.

I made the necessary changes to create a new life for myself and although it took work and I have to take precautions and be sensible, when it all goes well, it's so **worth it**!

Crossing the Road

Regardless if I am wearing my mask or not, before I cross a busy road, I try to find a spot that has clean air, then take a breath and hold it and then slowly let it out as I walk across the road. This way I am limiting the fumes I am breathing in from passing cars.

These days I do this without thinking and notice I am still slowly blowing out air even after I've crossed the road and I am walking down the street.

Tip...If you have young children, you could make it a game and teach them how to do it and that way it may help to limit the amount of diesel and petrol fumes they inhale.

DRIVING

It took me a few times to recognize that serious breathing issues were being brought on by either a truck that was in front of me and its exhaust was blowing toward my vehicle, or travelling behind cars that were blowing smoke or strong fumes and high traffic in general.

My breathing was being affected even though I had my windows up and my air-conditioning on recycled air. The fumes still got into the cabin of my vehicle and caused me immediate and at times serious breathing issues that could take many days to recover from.

Due to this being an extremely serious trigger, I do all I can to NOT drive when or where there is high traffic. If I have to drive somewhere in a built-up area, I will try to do it on a weekend or at night.

Even driving at night or weekends, I still need to be vigilant as I learnt not to underestimate how serious petrol and diesel fumes can impact on my breathing.

Dirt roads, I try to avoid them and if I can't, I usually drive very slowly to limit dust fluffing up and coming into my van. When such issues arise, I will implement my Plan of Action to reduce having breathing issues.

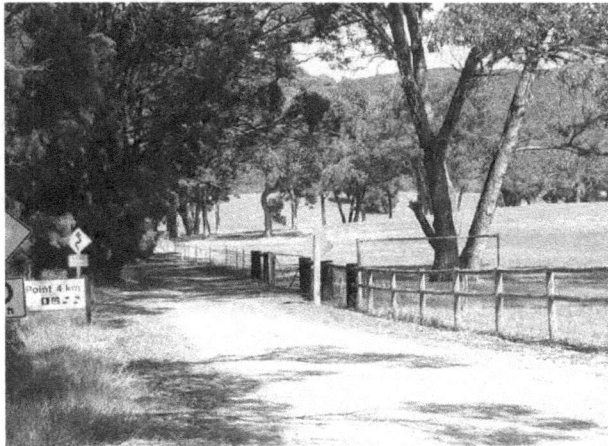

Roadworks can also be extremely challenging in regard to dust and if there is asphalting or taring happening then I put my Plan of Action in place and would pull over and put on my mask and use my medical air or oxygen depending on what I have packed in my van. The fact you usually have to drive slowly past roadworks means the fumes from other cars and the equipment used to fix or create the roads can also impact on my breathing, so I always have my windows up and I will turn on recycle-air in my van or turn it off.

Cab / Uber / Taxi

Until such time as being fragrant free is 'trendy', I believe you are going to have to contend with smells of all kinds in these vehicles. I have tried hiring upmarket cars but the driver still wore aftershave. I always have my small oxygen tank with me if I am in the city or built-up areas when using cabs and I cannot wind down the window because it lets other car fumes in!

It's such a conundrum and I recall I was on my way back to my van and only had a small distance to travel. I had a small amount of oxygen left in my small carry tank but I knew I had my large full medical air tank back at my van and another full small tank of oxygen. I always carried good supply when travelling. Sadly, the Uber driver had very strong aftershave, so I was using my oxygen and my hand fan and we ended up being caught in an unexpected traffic jam with lots of trucks around us and I was not able to wind down the window due to all the fumes outside. I tried to remain calm but he could hear I was struggling and in trouble, so he went up on the curb and into the emergency lane and got me back to my van where I immediately used my medical air. Suffice to say I survived, however it was extremely stressful and very scary.

Cruising – Ships

I have been on cruises prior to getting RADS and recall how narrow the corridors were and that everyone dressed up for dinner each night wearing perfume and aftershave and it would linger for long periods down the hall ways, in the stairwells and the lift. I could also smell when the room attendant had been in to make up my room and that was pre RADS! So as much as I would love to go on another cruise, I have decided, at this point in time, I'll just hold off for now. Maybe one day there will be a cruise ship that follows the lead of companies who are implementing scent/fragrant free environments and how cool would that be!

Plane

When I did fly, I called the airline about a week early and explained that I had RADS and described what it was. They were very understanding. I asked if I could board LAST because then people are not walking past me with fresh perfume on. Then I asked if I could get off FIRST, so I did not have to be subjected to fresh fumes from people re-spraying. I also asked if they could provide the little cart to drive me to the baggage area and save me being exposed to all the scents from people at the airport and the smells coming from the perfume shops etc. I also asked if I could take my small 5kg oxygen tank on board and they needed a letter from my specialist, which he kindly provided.

The airline went above and beyond that day for me and also blocked the seats either side of me. I was so grateful and very appreciative. Even with all the above in place, the person who sat in front of me began reading a newspaper and each time he turned a page the ink smell wafted over to me. So, I put my

Plan of Action into place and gargled some water and then discretely spat it into my empty bottle and used my hand fan to fluff the smell away and put the little air-conditioning button above me on full blast to also help propel clean air toward me and it all worked.

VERY IMPORTANT

Prior to having my small oxygen tank and just having masks, I did something without thinking as I had done it many times prior to getting RADS. I walked outside from the airport terminal with my mask on and crossed the road and waited for my ride. I was only across the road for a short time when I became overwhelmed very quickly by all the fumes from cars and buses going past that I began gasping for air and could feel my airways closing FAST. Tears ran down my face and I was terrified because I was running out of air and I could not speak, so I ran onto the road waving franticly.

Thankfully my friend overtook everyone else on the road and swung the passenger door open and pulled me in and turned the air-conditioner on high and sped off. It took me some time to settle my breathing and I ended up with extremely sore lungs due to the fumes I had inhaled. It was very traumatic and a life-threatening situation. Who would of thought?

My new strategy these days would be to wait inside the terminal away from people and the doors, with my mask on and oxygen on hand if needed. I would wait until my ride is at the curb with the door open and ready. I would speak to them on my phone and let them know that I will be holding my breath when I walk out to them, so I won't be speaking. I would then hold my breath calmly until I am safely in the car.

Public Transport – Bus

Due to the unpredictability of my condition and the fact a bus is a closed environment and I cannot stop people getting on the bus who may be wearing scented products, makes it very problematic and high risk for me. So, at this time, I do not use them.

Public Transport – Ferry

When I have used the large ferry, I explain to the staff that I have RADS and to limit my exposure to fumes, could I drive on first and get out my car and go upstairs inside the lounge before the rest of the cars drive on. They agreed and have always been understanding and very helpful. I take my small oxygen tank with me and sit away from people inside the lounge and if I go outside, I am careful not to be standing where the flue emits the smoke from the diesel.

Due to getting on first, means I also depart first and that's excellent! It's all about avoiding fumes and triggers!

Public Transport – Train

Due to the unpredictability of my RADS and the fact a train is a closed environment and I cannot stop people getting on the train who may be wearing scented products, makes it very problematic and high risk for me. So, at this time, I do not use them.

Travel to a City or Built-Up Areas

If I need to go to a city, then having my van means I can leave the night before and drive at night to minimize the fumes and pollution from trucks, cars and industry in and around the city.

I have stayed in a caravan park close to the city but I was exposed to fumes wafting out of the laundry room near the bathroom facility and some people sit around smoking. So, I park in a friend's mum's driveway as she is close to the city and I leave early to head to a small local swimming pool and have a shower there. I always hold my breath as I walk past the pool area due to chlorine being a strong trigger. So far, I have been in and out early and all was ok.

In my experience, driving in high traffic with diesel and petrol fumes can be extremely challenging and when I've been in the city, the tall buildings can trap the fumes and somehow, they usually find a way into my van. So, having my medical air tank in the vehicle with me and putting the tube under the chin of my cloth mask has been a great help.

Now if I have to drive to the other side of town I will only drive up at night or on the weekend to avoid all these issues and I may drive around built-up areas, even if it takes longer.

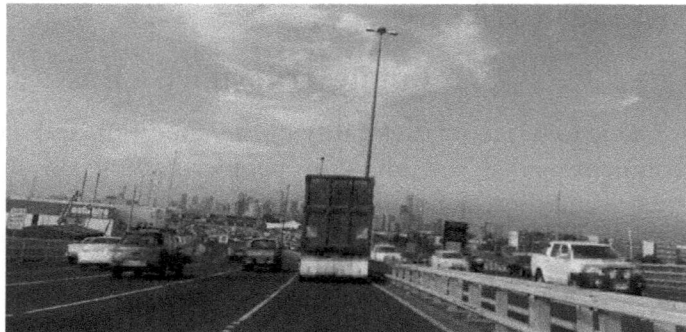

Vehicle – Campervan / Motorhome

If you are buying a second-hand van then you may need to check if people smoked in it or if it has ever had any "mildew or mould" etc. Also, if it has carpet or had pets in it, you may smell the dander and that may be an issue. If it is a "pop-top" then check the canvas for any signs of mould and if it has curtains, they may need to be replaced or washed to remove any past detergent smells.

Tip: Having a wind-up air vent has been a huge help in circulating air into my van at night however it can allow fine dust or smoke in. In regard to the dust,

I made a dust catcher out of a scarf that I folded in half and stitched. I hold it up on the roof by velcro and it does a good job filtering and limiting fine dust into my van through the roof air vent. (picture below) I also made sheer curtains to limit dust coming into my van from my sliding and back doors. (picture below)

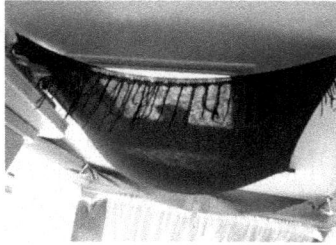

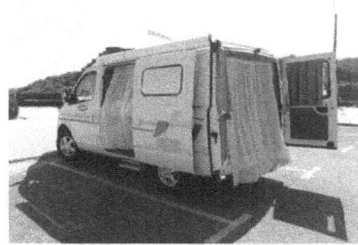

If you purchase a new van/motorhome it may take a few months (or longer) for the "new" smell to leave. I had to wash the curtains in vinegar and bi carb soda and wipe the cupboards out every few days with peppermint or eucalyptus oil as well as air the whole camper van for many weeks. I had to paint the pine timber in the cabinetry as it was off-gassing and causing me breathing issues. I also placed tubs of bi-carb soda in all the cupboards to try to absorb the new smell.

WARNING: I had my first van for 2.5 years and loved it but the battery in the back under my bed was not an AGM and as previously mentioned, it leaked heaps of sulphur dioxide fumes through my mattress and it could have killed me. I was not able to drive or sleep in it without experiencing major breathing issues, even months later. The sulphur smell leached into all the rubber seals, plastic dash, floor and wooden cabinetry. So, it's a good idea to check your battery and also make sure it is not placed over the top of the air holes! The whole van had to be written off, so having good insurance cover was paramount.

Tip...I have a strap between my front seats where I securely strap my medical air or small oxygen tank. It's secure and close by if I need to have un-contaminated air while I am on the road. It's been a life-saver for me.

Having a Van / Motorhome has enabled me to:-

Pack up fast if there is a pending issue (i.e. smoke from fires) and get away from the smell and knowing I have somewhere safe to sleep and enough clothes, water and food etc. to live ok for a number of days gives me great peace of mind. Extreme temperatures can cause me breathing issues, so when it is extremely cold in winter or blistering hot in summer, I can pack up and take off to a more suitable climate.

If I go away on holidays I can stay in my van, as many of the motels I have tried are not RADS friendly due to their cleaning chemicals or detergents they use to wash their linen or the carpet etc.

If I visit family and friends overnight, it's great to know I have my van to sleep in if their home has any triggers.

Vehicle – Cars

Initially, I had a sedan however, after getting RADS, I had occasions where I had to sleep in it and quickly realized a wagon or SUV type car or something I was able to comfortably lay down and sleep in, would have been extremely helpful.

Keeping your vehicle clean and limited dust is also really helpful. Cleaning with hot or warm water and either ask someone else to vacuum or make sure you wear good masks when cleaning and allow time for dust to settle before getting back in.

Once I had my car professionally cleaned and remembered to ask the cleaners to NOT use any chemicals and no air fresheners.

Unless I am driving in the mountains, or near the beach with a great breeze, I usually keep my windows up and have re-cycled air on in my vehicle, as I do not want to pull in air from outside, especially when I am in traffic.

Having an activated carbon cabin air filter fitted to your vehicle can be helpful in reducing and trapping dangerous contaminates and replacing the car's air conditioner filter yearly may also help.

It can be a difficult time when something that should be exciting, like buying a new car or another car, can be a mine-field of health issues for some people with RADS and other sensitivities. Buy new and you have the "new car smell" to contend with, buy second-hand and you have to check for smells like; mould, cigarette smoke, deodorizers, perfume etched into fabric car seats etc.

TIP….If I am out in the countryside and I wind my windows down to get lovely fresh air, I need to be mindful of dust and smells from freshly cut hay etc. that may affect my breathing. So, you need to be careful even when it all "looks" nice and safe outside.

Vehicles – Convertible

I tried riding in my cousin's convertible but we only travelled to the end of the street and had to turn around and go home as I was having severe breathing issues from the fumes from other vehicles and pollution in the air.

Vehicle – Disability Tag

An application for a vehicle disability tag is worth investigating. I was approved for a Disability Tag due to having breathing issues, when just trying to walk through car parks to get to a shop or an appointment. On one occasion due to so many fumes in the car park, I didn't even make it to the doors of the shopping center and ended up in hospital.

Having a Disability Tag has been a big help to me. I can now park right near the door of any appointment or store and this has greatly reduced the fumes I breathe in when exiting my van. It's also extremely helpful if I need to take my small oxygen tank with me, as it's less distance I have to carry it.

Vehicle – Fuel stations

Petrol, diesel and oil are all very strong triggers for me, so if you don't have a partner or friend with you at the fuel station and you need fuel, then here is what I do to limit my exposure: -

- ✓ Fill up in the evening or very early in the morning, when it is not busy and there is no queue.
- ✓ Before pulling in, look for a pump that does not have diesel or petrol spilt on the ground because if you stand on it, it may soak into the sole of your shoes and then you will carry that smell into your vehicle.
- ✓ I always wear my heavy-duty mask when filling up my van and depending on the breeze situation, I might also wrap a scarf around my face to help lessen breathing in fumes.
- ✓ I always tear some paper towel and put it on my hand as I lift up the pump, or I will put on a plastic glove if I have some in the van. (some pumps have fuel on the handle and once it's on your skin it's very hard to get off and have caused me serious breathing issues.)
- ✓ Work out where the breeze is blowing and turn your face and body away from the fumes from the pump.
- ✓ When going in to pay, I throw away the glove or paper towel but leave my mask on until I get to the door and I pull it down so the teller can see my face. I pull my mask up to walk back to my van and usually hold my breath until I am inside my van.

TIP… I ignore any people who stare at me. Those poor folks are breathing in all those fumes.

Vehicles – Hepa filters

As previously mentioned, having special filters fitted to your car's air inlet vent etc. can make a difference to the air quality that comes into the cabin of your vehicle. They vary in price and some people have found them to be very good in helping to reduce dust and pollution etc. coming into your vehicle.

Vehicles – Hire Car or Vehicles

I didn't even think about this until I had to hire a car and was not able to sit in it due to the smell of the cleaning products they had used. The company was wonderful and they took the very next car in (an upgrade) and cleaned it with warm water and nothing else and I was good to go! If you need to hire a car it might be worth calling a day or so before and let them know about your sensitivities.

Vehicles – Jet Ski

I have not ridden a jet ski since my injury and I would think that as long as the wind was blowing toward you, then that may blow the fumes from the jet ski away from you. It's not something I have tried post RADS but I sure hope I can one day because I have ridden them in the past and they were great fun.

Vehicles – Motor Bike

I had motorbikes for a long time and since having RADS I had to stop riding due to not being able to find any mask strong enough that would protect my airways from the fumes and pollution when riding. I am still trying to find a helmet or mask or create a breathing device that will work, stay tuned!

Vehicle – What I Keep in My Van

Masks, small oxygen tank, water bottles, hand fan, plastic gloves, serviettes, scarf, change of clothes, chewing gum, plastic rain coat cover, pen and paper for writing a note if I can't speak and an air horn in the event I can't talk and I require immediate help or I am in trouble.

Keeping a quilt, blankets, pillow or mattress in the back is also really helpful for any emergency situations where I may have to leave quickly (i.e. bush fire), home emergency (i.e. gas leak), burn-off from local farmers etc.

I have emergency contact details in my phone and I also have a print out in my phone sleeve.

SHOPPING

Local Shopping

Where I now live there is a short main street not far away which is opposite the ocean and on good air days, it can blow a lovely breeze down the street and dissipate fumes from cars. On these good days, I can have a wander around going into many shops. If my Chief Air Assessor notices any smells coming out the front door of a shop, I will put my Plan of Action in place and move away or cross the road away from it and if needed gargle or do what I need to manage my breathing.

Sometimes I get caught going into a shop I think is initially "safe" for me and the deeper I get inside I begin to have a reaction, so I immediately leave. This is usually due to air fresheners or those sticks in oil that are on some counter tops.

Remaining calm knowing I have my Plan of Action is a great comfort and enables me to successfully navigate my way through any situation. Having practiced it for many years, each step and option comes second nature now.

Shopping Centers

Soon after my injury, I had a very severe breathing issue just trying to walk through a car park to the doors of the shopping center. Unbeknown to me, the cars pulling in and out of the parks were releasing diesel and petrol fumes all around me which caused me serious respiratory distress. It was very traumatic and I ended up in hospital. Who would have thought, just trying to walk to the doors of a shopping center, could place me in a potentially life-threatening situation?

Once I realized it was the car fumes that caused me to have such a serious reaction, I researched which shops were open at night and I would go late in the evenings when there were less people and fewer cars.

These days, having a Disability Tag means I can park right near the main entry and I sometimes wear my mask when leaving my car if I can smell fumes or taste dust in the air.

Depending on how I feel and how long I am going to be and exactly where I am going inside the center, I will sometimes take my small oxygen tank in a shopping trolley. Once inside the center I check the air quality and depending on how busy it is and the smell and taste of the air, I may or may not leave my mask on. More often I will leave it on because I sometimes end up with sore lungs the next day after being at a shopping center where I'm exposed to new and different smells.

I also now know what shops to avoid walking past like nail shops, soap shops, candle shops, hairdressing salons and if I walk into any shops that have boxes of detergent out front, I hold my breath and try to avoid being anywhere near them.

While some shops can be great one day and don't give me breathing issues, I could go another time and have problems breathing. It's very hit and miss. There may be renovation works or cleaning of air-conditioning units, shops getting refitted etc. let alone people wearing fragrances. All these anomalies can have an impact on the air quality and my breathing and rather than stress, I remain calm because I know what I need to do if there is an issue and follow my Plan of Action.

Shopping Online and Home Delivery

Prior to moving from suburbia, I was highly reactive and unable to leave my home without experiencing severe breathing issues, so thank goodness for the internet and home delivery because I ordered all my food shopping online and had it delivered.

The super powers of RADS amazed me that I could even smell the delivery guy's aftershave through the cracks in my closed front door. He would leave it on the step outside and I wouldn't go out until the wind had blown the scent away.

Supermarket

The detergent isle in most supermarkets can cause me significant respiratory issues. My solution is to avoid them and if I can't send a friend to get what I need, then I ask the staff and I have always found them to be helpful. I also hold my breath anytime I walk past that isle or if they have detergent displays. The pet food isle can sometimes cause me breathing issues too, so I avoid that isle unless I need something for my pup and then I might just hold my breath and I'm usually out of harm's way by the time I need more air.

I have tried to use the "do it yourself" checkouts and sadly I got caught out with a lady who stood next to me wearing a very strong perfume. I had an immediate reaction and grabbed my purse coughing and left my groceries. The attendant saw what happened and sent someone to check on me, which was very nice. They put my frozen groceries back and kept the rest of my shopping for another time when I was ready to go back.

My solution is I now shop in the middle of the day or late at night when there are limited people inside. I no longer use those "do it yourself" check outs and always take a trolley and use the normal check outs where someone serves you because I have more room to move away from people if they are wearing any scented products and I can place the trolley between them and me.

Some staff at my local supermarket know me and after a few conversations they now understand why I have days I might wear my mask and others when I don't need to. Some staff will look at me when I don't have my mask on and say "It's a good air day today for you?" and I smile and say "sure is!"

LOOKING FOR ACCOMMODATION

I had to look for a room to rent while I was in the transition period while my house was being built and that presented new problems I didn't foresee. Over the years I have spoken to many people with RADS who have been faced with the same challenges when searching for rental properties or rooms to rent.

Each time I was inside a potential rental property I could smell a range of the following:- Cleaning chemicals or laundry odors, carpet fibers, mould, scented products wafting from the bathroom, room deodorizers or pet dander.

I knew within moments of being inside if I would be triggered and I was becoming quite desperate after seeing nine rooms that were all unsuitable. Some were right next to bathrooms or the laundry room or they omitted strong odours. I was horrified to find one place stunk of mould, so I walked in and straight out the door.

I printed a number of flyers and left them in letter box's asking if anyone had a room for rent. Sadly, I had no replies.

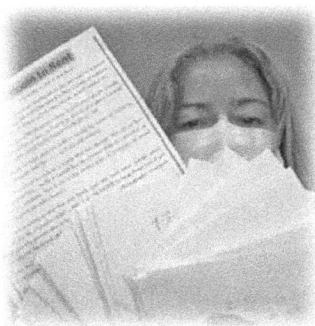

I tried staying in a caravan park but the only room left was behind a fuel station and I had to leave due to the smell of fumes entering the unit I was in.

I ended up sleeping in my car (this was before I had my van) and that was very challenging and a difficult time however I felt I had no other option and fortunately soon after I struck gold when I went and saw a room for rent that was perfect!

My flat mate didn't like chemicals and was very neat and tidy and he wasn't fussed about *not* wearing any scented products or changing washing products. In fact, he went above and beyond by re-showering if I could smell chlorine on him if he walked in the house after being at the local pool. I was so grateful and appreciated this so much!

He has remained a good friend to this day and inspired me to buy my campervan. I was extremely relieved and very grateful to have a safe, clean non-triggering roof over my head and sharing with someone who was thoughtful and accommodating of my RADS. Pretty darn amazing really!

Creating an environment in your home that is free from toxins, fragrances, chemicals and alike, isn't a fast and easy thing to achieve. I had marketing so entrenched in my mind from years of television commercials suggesting my home should smell like roses to be inviting and clean or my toilet is much cleaner if some chemically enhanced product made the water a different color, that I overlooked the chemicals they may be omitting. Now living with extreme sensitivities, my sense of smell and taste ramped up to what felt like super human levels, so I began having serious breathing issues from a multitude of toxins just being at home.

This is why creating a safe room is so important. Somewhere to rest and heal while clearing out toxins, chemicals and fragrances from inside your home. It was a long slow process doing it on my own, however once it was achieved, I only had to think about who came into my home, what odors they brought with them and what I would be faced with once I walked out my front door. Over the early years of having RADS I had to make changes to reduce my triggers inside my home and at the house where I was renting a room. Through trial and error and the process of elimination, I was able to achieve good results by making the following changes.

Books and Paper

The smell from either the ink or the paper of some new books can cause me quite strong breathing issues. I place the offending item outside undercover and it can take a number of days or weeks for the pages to "de-smell" and air out. If you have ordered my book as a physical book, then you may have to also air it out.

TIP... if you have old books on a shelf, they may collect fine dust and the pages can smell very strong. If you do de-dust them, then maybe once that is done you could try laying material on top of the books to smother some of the smell and keep the dust off.

Bathroom – Cleaning

I have a glass bottle that I put orange peel in and then I pour white vinegar in and seal it. This creates a nice gentle orange smell and it is used to clean all my bathrooms and they sparkle and cause me no breathing issues. If just vinegar was used, it would be too overwhelming for me, so with the orange smell it's nice. You can also use lemon or mandarin peel instead or with the orange peel.

Bathroom – Personal

Perfume and Aftershave – I immediately had to stop wearing perfume which wasn't too difficult for me as I only wore it on special occasions. For some people I speak with, it's part of their daily routine, so it's a bigger adjustment. Removing the physical bottles from my home needed to be done to stop the lingering smell. It amazed me just how strong and long a fume would last and how far the smell would carry.

The frequency I smell perfume or aftershave on others, out walking, jogging or just at the supermarket etc. leads me to think, for many, it's used regularly. As previously explained, the breathing issues I experience when exposed to fumes from various perfume, aftershave or deodorants etc. can range from mild to life-threatening, so I do all I can to avoid fumes when I am out.

Even if I wear masks when I am out, I can still smell a strong perfume or aftershave through my mask, so I always **remove** and replace that mask **asap** because the fume can contaminate it. I am always glad I had my mask on, because my thinking is, the mask has at least absorbed some of the initial fume, so I only get the remnants and it means I may only be hypersensitive and have breathing issues for a short time, instead of days or weeks.

When I smell strong fragrances on parents who pass me pushing strollers, nursing babies or holding a toddlers' hand, I just feel so sad.

On one occasion, I was at a lookout with a wonderful fresh breeze blowing and I could hear a man in the distance coughing and then I *smelt* why! They were still coming down stairs behind me and thank goodness the breeze was blowing most of her fume away from me. I asked her to stop on the stairs for a moment while I put on my mask and packed my camera away. I explained her perfume was VERY strong and I needed to leave. She thankfully complied and the look on her partners face was priceless, as he nodded in agreement with me and rolled his eyes in-between coughing. I quickly removed my mask for a moment, faced the breeze and took a big breath of clean air, put my mask back on and held my breath as I calmly maneuvered around them nodding with thanks for waiting. I walked up the stairs, along the short path slowly exhaling and reached my van. I took off my jumper and mask and put them in a plastic bag to contain the smell and then gargled and spat some clean water. It's amazing, when you think you are in a safe situation standing on a lookout, on the edge of a cliff, with amazing clean air all around and then this happens!

Please check the internet for information in regard to what chemicals are used in various perfumes and other everyday products like washing powder, fabric softeners etc.

Showering – I ensured I had an "outdoor shower" in my new home, especially for when I am trying new hair products. It's been fantastic in summer and allows me to try different products and not contaminate my inside bathroom, in the event of a failed product.

Deodorants - Initially I used an unscented roll-on deodorant however after more research into non-chemical deodorants, I have tried numerous brands over the years. Then I came across the one I am using at the moment and I am thrilled, as it's been working great for over twelve months and not one breathing issue!

Not only is it all natural, it also has a choice of four different lovely fresh aromas and it's now something I look forward to using each morning because having RADS meant I had to remove fragrances from my life. The one I am using at the moment smells like citrus with a dash of sunshine, making me feel bright and happy when I smell it.

Soap – I have been using the yellow old fashion bar of soap ever since having RADS, as I didn't want to keep contaminating myself with trying different soaps, when this one worked. Now and then I might use a goat's milk soap but I don't get too adventurous because it's just not worth the breathing issues they can cause me. So, for now I just stick with what works for me.

Conditioner – I keep trying lots of different brands and the best so far seems to be non-chemical conditioners with a coconut base.

Hair Gel – A friend wanted to use hair gel, so we went and tested some and the ones that gave me the least issues were those that smelt like coconut.

Body Lotion – I use organic coconut oil and that's it.

Hair Dye – I used to use a no ammonia hair dye and it was a bit of an ordeal doing it myself. I did it outside and wash it out under my outside shower and never use the conditioner they provide as it's usually overpowering, so I use my own no fragrant conditioner. Having done it myself for a number of years, I am very fast. I have been told of some natural hair dyes coming onto the market, so that's great. I did recently find a no ammonia salon and had my hair cut and colored without any breathing issues, so that was wonderful and a great experience just to be out in a salon and not have any breathing problems. Yay!

Toilet paper – Who would have thought that toilet paper could cause breathing issues? Well it did for me! Some have very strong bleach or perfume, so it took me a while to find a brand that didn't cause me breathing issues. I especially noticed the strong smell when I would open up the cupboard where it was kept.

Nails– I file and cut my own nails and only recently (on a windy day) I painted my toe nails outside while wearing my good mask and was ok as there was a strong breeze. I don't have any nail varnish remover as it's a terrible trigger for me, so once this wears off, I might just paint a bit more. At one stage I did put all my nail polish and removers out in my shed in a plastic bag and I put that inside a plastic container but the smell leached into it, so I threw the whole thing away. I get amazed at the super powers of having RADS!

Carpet

I notice that certain carpet can cause breathing issues for me. I think it is mostly due to the fact carpet needs to be vacuumed and can hold dust. I get amazed that I can smell the carpet fiber. Unfortunately, the blowing out of the vacuum cleaner seems to fluff up very fine dust and fibers and that can cause me huge breathing problems.

If you have carpet that you cannot pull up or get rid of, then maybe have someone else vacuum it for you and leave the room or home while it is being done and don't come back until the fine dust has settled. For me this could be an hour or more.

When I was trying to walk into display homes, the new carpet smell was especially bad for me and gave me severe breathing issues where I would have to promptly leave the home. I couldn't stay inside long enough to identify if it was some kind of chemical omitting from it or the fibers. Due to this being such a big issue for me, when I built my home, I made sure it had no carpet and all engineered highly polished concrete floors throughout with no resin/epoxy.

TIP ...Smothering carpet with clean sheets (that were washed in non-fragrant/chemical product) was a big help to me prior to getting my van. I would smother the carpet in a little room I once rented and I also smothered it when I stayed away and it worked great to contain the smell from the carpet. A number of people I have spoken to with RADS have had their carpet removed and it's made a big difference in helping them to breathe easier in their home. Others are using sheets to smother and cover their bedroom carpet, which also helps.

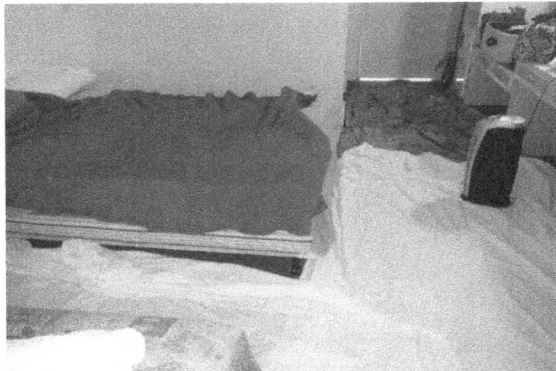

Clothing

I keep a plastic bag and spare sweater and top in my van in the event I have hugged someone hello and they had perfume or aftershave on their clothing. I can quickly change and put the smelly clothing in the plastic bag to wash at home later.

Tip..If washing detergents and fabric softeners cause you breathing issues, then you may need to re-wash all your clothing and bedding. I wash mine in either dissolved bi-carb soda or an eco-sensitive liquid with a splash of white vinegar (as a fabric softener) and no my clothes don't smell like vinegar... amazing hey!

Cooling

At this time, I just use ceiling fans as I do not need an air-conditioner and I made sure I had security screens installed on doors and windows, so I was able to have them open most days to allow good air flow.

If however I did get one, I would be very selective making sure it had good hepa filters and not get anything that emits ozone or has an ionizer.

I believe some units will draw air from outside and this could be a problem if the outside air was compromised with smoke or other harmful pollutants. So, if I was ever thinking of purchasing one, I would do some investigative homework first.

When I have been at a friend's home who has an air-conditioning unit, I felt fine as well as feeling good in our large shops in summer when they are running their air conditioning. Again, it can be a bit hit and miss because I have walked into smaller shops and had to immediately walk out due to what felt like dust being blown from their air-conditioning unit.

Curtains

I tried to hang curtains that had "block out" on the back and I had immediate and severe respiratory distress. So, I asked a friend to wash them in the bath with vinegar and non-fragrant soapy water and hung them on the line for three days to air dry. When they were re-hung back in the room, they still stank of the block out smell and gave me breathing issues. I was amazed at how strong the smell was. I took them back and was given a full refund being told, it was not uncommon that they omit a strong smell like that.

Once I moved, I had backing curtains especially made that did NOT have any block out on them. Amazingly they cost me more money? Go figure!

I suggest if you have RADS, to not overlook the dust that curtains can hold and fluff off when they are open or closed. It's a good idea to wash all curtains to remove dust, especially if you are creating a safe room that has curtains in it. Even taking them down can trigger some people, so wearing a good mask might be a good idea before hand washing them. It may also be a good idea to regularly wipe down venetian type blinds to help limit dust.

Tip...I had off-white "scrim" curtains made for my home to help catch dust blowing through my windows and sliding doors and WOW how good do they work! After a few months I was surprised when they were hand washed to see how brown and dirty the water was. They were a good investment indeed. Due to them working so well, I made some for my sliding door in my van and the back too and they also work great!

Footwear

A number of shoe stores can be very difficult for me to just walk into and this is usually due to the strong smell of rubber and plastic.

I have to also be very careful about what shoes I purchase because the smell can contaminate my clothing if it's in close proximity in my wardrobe. I put most new shoes out in my garage until the "new" smell has gone and some I have had to give away, as the smell just wouldn't go.

It's all trial and error and it's great when it works out!

Uhh the Super Powers of having RADS
Use your Super Power for Good ☺

Heating

My home in suburbia had ducted heating and for me it was a nightmare. It took me many weeks of broken sleep and severe breathing issues to finally work out it was my ducted heating. It had a timer and when I was asleep it would come on through the night and fluff up fine dust and cause me to wake up gasping as my airways would start closing. I was so sleep-deprived and having such severe attacks, I wasn't joining the dots. Eventually once I realized it was the ducted heating, I tried covering the vents with two pairs of panty-hose. That didn't work and I was still having breathing issues, so I had to turn it off and I slept with a knitted hat and scarf on for the next few months.

At one stage I tried getting my old radiant heater out of my garage but when I put it on the dust on, the elements gave me immediate breathing issues. I have tried being in a home that had a Coonara/wood heater, where the wood is put into a cast iron box and there is a flue going up to the roof. Although I was assured there would be no smell, each time the door was open to put more wood in, a puff of smoke would filter out and cause me breathing issues.

My friends have a gas heater behind glass and my breathing has been good when I am close to it and I have never had any breathing issues. They also have a gas oven and whenever they have it on, I can smell gas, so there is a gas leak which I have told them about. Oh the Super Powers of RADS!

Please be **<u>very</u> careful** of any leaking gas connections and always call your gas company if you can smell gas. If you have inhaled gas, it's sensible to go straight to hospital so they can check if you have carbon monoxide poisoning. Don't wait, act on it asap because it can be very dangerous and life threatening.

I do not have breathing issues without cause, it's always triggered from something, so I trust my awesome Chief Air Assessor. Trusting and listening to my body when it gives me the signs that something is not right, happens automatically after many years of practice.

Although my new home has hydronic heating, which is supposed to be good for not blowing heat, I still have breathing issues when it's on, so when I turn it off, it can be extremely cold in winter … until… (and thank you to the person who invented these) I tried an electric throw rug and I could then sit on my sofa with the door slightly open to let the lovely clean cool air come in and not freeze. I love my new electric throw rug and it would be a very brave person who ever tried to remove it from my sofa! Funny how those little things can bring you so much pleasure.

Heat Bag

I can't use a heat bag with wheat in it as I found out, it gives me breathing issues. So, I made one with rice in it and it seems to work ok.

Kitchen – Cooking Smells

After getting RADS I have become chemically sensitive to some foods. I can no longer have any cinnamon, pepper, chili or anything spicy or hot because when I have tried the tiniest amount, I have immediate and severe breathing issues. I also avoid being in a room where chili is being cooked. I must also have the extraction fan on if I am cooking fish or my airways can react.

Kitchen – Dishwasher

At this time, I am unaware of a commercial non-toxic dishwasher tablet on the market, so until one comes out, I wash all my dishes by hand with an Eco detergent. Going back to the old fashion way of doing dishes can have some positives like:-

1/ You are not subjecting your lungs and airways to the smells some tablets omit when opening the packet or sachet.
2/ The smell won't leach into the cupboard where they are placed if the packet is open.
3/ You won't be breathing in any potentially contaminated steam/air when opening the door of the dishwasher.
4/ Usually people have a good old chat and communicate while doing the dishes.
5/ You could save money not having to pay for washing tablets and buy an eco-detergent to hand wash them instead.
6/ You could perfect the art of negotiating i.e. who gets to wash, dry or put away and just learning how to wash and dry dishes, I think, is a good life lesson for many.
7/ Save on power costs, as you are not running your dishwasher.

8/ You could have dishes washed, dried and put away before some machines have even started the rinse cycle.

Kitchen – Flies and Spiders

Since having RADS, I went and purchased a butterfly catcher and I use that to catch flies and spiders and then release them outside. I think I've released a few flies with a headache! This is great for children to also learn to do and means there is zero omission and no fumes!

Kitchen – Paper Towels

Be mindful there are certain brands of paper towel that may omit a smell like bleach. It took me a while to figure it out and when I did, I now wrap them in a plastic bag and the smell is contained. It was especially strong in a closed environment like a cupboard and in my van.

Kitchen – Rubbish Bags

I found scented rubbish bags are a trigger and give me breathing issues, so I buy the basic unscented type.

Laundry

Learning to live with RADS, I soon realized I had to throw out all my washing detergent and all my fabric softener's as they were one of the big culprits giving me ongoing breathing issues. They had to be put into plastic bags like toxic waste in a bin outside my home and it was imperative I did not touch it. If you feel your detergents may be causing you issues and you can get someone else to remove it and put it in plastic bags out of your home, that's great. If not, then put gloves on or pull plastic bags over your hands to protect them and wear a good mask or two!

My whole laundry (walls and floors) and washing machine had to be wiped down with hot water numerous times in an effort to remove the smell. I didn't use any other cleaning products because I needed to identify when the chemical smells had gone and if you use oils like peppermint or eucalyptus at that early stage, it may mask over the chemical smell.

Unfortunately, the chemical smell from the washing products had leached into my paint work, so I had to have the laundry door open to outside for many months and I placed a towel at the bottom of the internal door, to keep the smell out of the rest of the house. Yes, it was that bad for me and if you have a similar reaction then you could try doing the same. I ran a few cycles of hot water and half a cup of white vinegar through my washing machine to help clear the chemicals and it seemed to work well cleaning my machine. Check with your manufacturer about the best way to clean your machine.

Not only were the chemicals in the laundry room, they were also in my clothes. Everything I was wearing was causing me triggers including the bed sheets and towels. I was triggering myself and I didn't realize it!

My clothes and bedding had been off-gassing these very strong fumes and I never knew this until I had the Super Powers of RADS. It was a big contributor in prolonging my coughing and breathing issues and I can't stress enough the importance for people to have a serious look at their laundry, bathroom and toilet products.

My solution was that I initially took out a weeks' worth of clothes I wore all the time and a set of sheets and towels and washed them in hot water with Bi-carb (or soapy water) and half a cup of white vinegar. Everything else went into garbage bags out the house and into the shed until I had time to re-wash it with the same as above. By the way, I found that white vinegar has been the best fabric softener I have ever used and there was no smell of vinegar! Seriously, none! My towels come up lovely and fluffy even after being out on a clothes line. I was so happy!

Tip...Rather than have to wait for a whole wash cycle, I just filled up the laundry sink with hot water, dissolved about four heaped table spoons of Bi-carb (or sometimes I used soapy water I made by swishing around a bar of plain soap in the water and then took out the bar and made sure there were no fragments of soap in the water or it will stick to your fabric) and about half a cup of white vinegar in the water and then hand washed the equivalent of a full load, then put it to one side in a bucket and then emptied the sink and filled it up with clean water and rinsed everything and hand squeezed the water out. Then I put it in my washing machine and set it to "spin" and spun the excess water out and hung it on the line or air rack to dry. This sped up the process and I could wash the equivalent to five loads in a very short time by doing it by hand. It's not that the items were dirty; I was just removing the smell from the old detergent or fabric softener. Some items I washed a couple of times but they still stunk of fabric softener, so I had to throw them away.

I no longer use my clothes dryer. Instead I air-dry everything on the line, so I pick a warm day. In winter I use an airing rack inside my home and my clothes are usually dry within a couple of days. For some who do use their clothes dryer, they place them in their garage and if that's not an option they ensure it is regularly wiped out and the lint filter is kept clean. Don't under estimate how noxious the residual smell from your laundry can be and how long it can last in certain flooring and walls.

I would rate my laundry room, washing detergent and fabric softener in the top of my list of items I needed to immediately change or clean out.

It's very much trial and error when trying to find a detergent that doesn't give you breathing issues. I initially used plain soap and made soapy water and put it into my machine with half a cup of vinegar and spent a lot of money trying lots of labelled "chemical free" or "fragrance free" detergents. I finally found a chemical free laundry liquid that worked great for me. Be mindful that just because a product may say it is "fragrance free", doesn't mean it is free from chemicals. Also, I always dilute my washing product in a bucket with a splash of vinegar and then pour that into my machine and it's been working great for me for years. I hope you find one that suits you.

It may also be a good idea to check how close your neighbors' clothesline is to your windows or doors as I have had significant breathing issues from scents invading my home from the neighbor hanging out their washing and the smell of strong fabric softener coming through my open windows. At a rental home I stayed in and in a room upstairs, I could smell the neighbor's fabric softener that wafted up from their clothes line and through my open window.

Once I identified why I was having the breathing issues, I just had to make sure I shut my door and windows when they did their washing.

Don't underestimate how far the smell of washing detergent and especially some fabric softeners can travel and what an impact it may have on your breathing.

New Clothing and Bedding

I wash all new clothing, underwear and bedding because a lot of it has "fire retardants" and who knows what other chemicals on them So, it's always best to wash everything before you have it on you or near you. I wash mine in either bi-carb or my special washing liquid and some white vinegar, then air them on the clothes line.

Newspaper and junk mail

The ink on newspapers are a big issue for me and especially when they are new. If a newspaper is on a table in an office or lounge room, then I have to either leave the room, or have the newspaper removed. When I have tried to move it myself, I have to hold my breath and I just use two fingers to pick it up and remove it. Then I must wash my fingers or I will continue to have breathing issues from the smell of the ink on my fingers. It's that strong to me!

If you are also sensitive to newspaper ink and someone in your home likes to read the newspaper, then maybe ask if they could read it outside and away from any windows to avoid the smell blowing in. Once finished, they would also need to wash their hands too or you may smell it when they are near you. Dispose of the newspaper outside of the home or in a concealed bag.

New Furniture and Beds

Formaldehyde has caused me serious breathing issues and I wasn't aware it can be in furniture and mattresses and so many other products. I purchased a lovely new bedroom suite and new mattress and tried to sleep on it 4 times over 1.5 years.

The first time I tried, I only lasted a few minutes and had to call the paramedics due to my airways closing very fast and I was in serious trouble. I immediately removed myself and waited many months and aired my bedroom every day until I tried to sleep on the bed again. When I did try, I had breathing issues and spat up blood, so I waited six months and even took some of the pieces outside on nice sunny days to air but when I tried to sleep the mattress, I still had breathing issues and blood. One and a half years later I paid an Air Quality Test company to come and take samples of the air in my bedroom and sure enough, my bedroom with all the new furniture and new mattress, was omitting disturbing levels of VOC (Volatile Organic Compounds) and formaldehyde. I contacted the furniture company and they agreed to collect all the furniture and gave me a refund. I tried to sleep in other rooms in my home but sadly I still had breathing issues.

This was the catalyst for me to purchase a campervan to sleep -in my driveway or by the ocean. I have aired my bedroom and house every day and night ever since (which has been nearly four years). Regretfully I still have issues when I try to sleep inside my home, however I do notice it is slowly getting better, so I am hopeful that whatever is still "gassing-off" will clear in the next twelve months.

TIP....I researched and found a local mattress company who make all their mattresses in-house with no formaldehyde, so I purchased a new mattress and a cast iron bed. Some people also purchase older second-hand furniture which can also work well. I found the internet helpful to locate these outlets and manufactures in my area and you could do the same.

Outside Yard

Due to the fact some lawn mowers and edge cutters are run on petrol and I know petrol fumes cause me major breathing issues, I put fake lawn in my backyard and made my front yard very low maintenance with some Australian native plants

If my neighbor's start their lawn mowers or edger's, then I come inside or get away from the fumes and I close my windows. If there are major works going on near my home (landscaping, road works) then I close my windows and maybe leave my home and go out for the day.

I know battery operated or electric lawn mowers or hand push ones may be useful however I still have issues from the strong smell of cut grass and dust.

Please also be mindful that blowers fluff up dust and other particles, as well as raking and sweeping, so doing these tasks might cause breathing issues for some.

A great solution has been getting an outside vacuum cleaner to suck up dust and leaves and still wearing a good mask is sensible if you do it. With dust being a very serious trigger for me, I do all I can to limit it in my life.

In regard to potting mix, it's always a really good idea to read the label, as some may contain ingredients that could create a serious trigger, so knowing this, I don't use it and will get someone else to get it, in the event anything needs to be re-potted. In fact, I won't go near the potting mix aisle at the local garden supply place due to the strong smell.

Even the smell of some healthy soil or dirt can cause me respiratory issues and the smell of new bark, some plants, bushes and some flowers. Products and items I would not have thought about, until I was near to them.

Knowing I have RADS, I went in search of a tall shrub that wouldn't give off much smell and would not drop a lot of leaves as I wanted to create a filter type block around my backyard to help limit smoke or air pollution. I decided on Lily Pilly's which are growing nicely and, in another year, I expect them to be quite a bit taller. I have cut them on the tops so they bush up more and become denser.

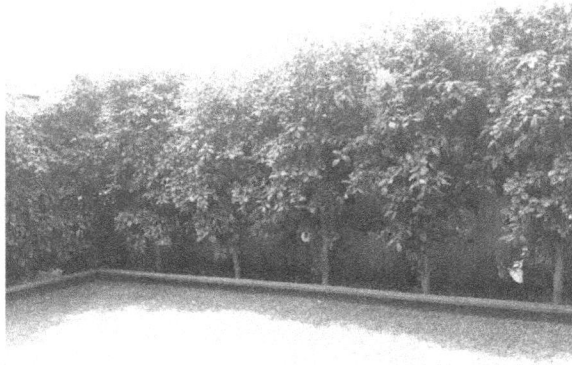

Paints

I went to great lengths and cost to ensure my home was painted with the latest No VOC (volatile organic compounds) paint available at that time. I think it may have had other chemicals in it that could have caused me breathing issues, so I had three rooms painted with three different paints to see if it made any difference. It didn't make any difference. In fact, for my situation the No VOC paint had no smell of paint (as I know it) but it did have some other smell I could not identify.

If anyone came into my home, they would say it had that "new house smell" which did not agree with my RADS. I feel it's definitely a matter of test and smell and feel how your breathing feels because we are all different and it may take weeks, months or in my case, years to try and figure out.

Pets

In regard to dogs, I had two gorgeous senior fur babies who were nine and fifteen and since having RADS I began experiencing breathing issues when they came close to me and I had no idea why, so I had to keep moving them back from me. Tragically they passed away within a short time after I was diagnosed and I missed them every single day.

After speaking to other pet owners who also have RADS, I soon realized I wasn't alone in regard to having occasional breathing issues if they were up close.

Having RADS can be very isolating and lonely and after having dogs my whole adult life, I decided six years was long enough living without a pet and since accomplishing a better quality of life I felt confident and ready for my beautiful puppy. I searched all over the internet to find the best fit pet for me and decided on a Poochie. She is the most adorable Poodle x Chihuahua and has brought so much joy and love into my world. The Poodle in her means she won't shed her fur and being part Chihuahua means she is little, so she will only produce a small amount of dog dander. Also, being a puppy, I knew I could train her to help limit triggering me by way of being covered up and wrapped up now and then and she's very content when I need to do it.

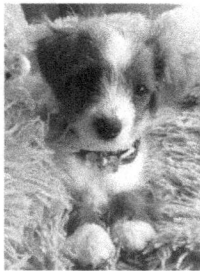

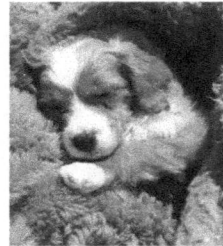

I believe some people think that when a dog is described as being "hypoallergenic" it means it won't cause asthma or breathing issues etc.

My understanding is that "hypoallergenic" means their fur is human like and won't shed like other breeds. Every dog has "dog dander" and it is a very fine dandruff dust that comes from the skin which is what can cause some people various health issues. Please check the internet yourself to verify this.

Although my puppy is a small breed, she still has dog dander and do the following to help minimize any impact on my breathing: -

In between washes and if I can detect any puppy/dog smell then I might put a little breathable jacket for summer on her and a warmer one for winter. This helps to smother any dander or fine dust from her skin and keeps it inside the jacket.

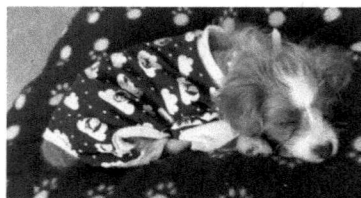

- When her jacket is off, I try not to fluff her fur too much when patting her.

- I try to refrain from having her up near my face, unless she has recently had a bath.

- Sometimes I will wrap her in a puppy blanket when I am holding her.

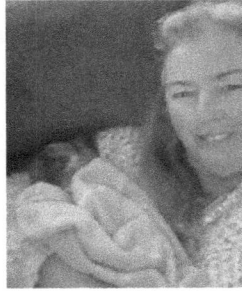

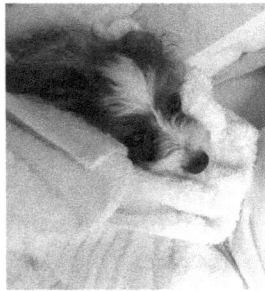

- I wash her as needed with unscented products.

- At bedtime my pup has her own bed nearby to mine and in eyesight and most mornings when I lift her up for a snuggle, she stays wrapped in her blanket until she does a morning yoga stretch.

- Her dog beds and blankets are all washed in my non-chemical washing product.

- My home is regularly mopped with microfiber mops to reduce any dog dander and dust.

- My pup has her own blankets she sits on if she is in my van. That way her smell is not all over my car seats or bedding.

- I also have throw rugs over my sofa, so if she does jump up on it, they can be easily washed.

Please Beware: - I read the back of the liquid flea and heart worm product whereby you just put a couple of drops on the neck. The packet explains to not breathe in the fumes etc. so I was trying to be very sensible especially due to having sensitivities and put my mask and gloves on and I did it outside. After a couple of hours of her running around and doing puppy stuff outside, she came and sat next to me and I immediately started to have breathing issues because I could still smell the liquid on her. I put clean gloves on and my good mask and washed the remainder off her. I then sat near the back door to get a clean breeze and used some of my medical air. Fortunately doing that helped to settle my airways and stop a further reaction.

So please don't underestimate the strength and toxicity of some treatments on the market for your pets as they may cause a trigger.

Also, I recently spoke with a lovely couple who had a very sick dog and they decided to try cleaning out all chemicals and fragrant products in their home and live as chemical free as possible to see if it would have any positive impact on their dog's health. For their specific situation, over time their dog's health improved dramatically and it's now received a clean bill of health from the vet. So, it's an important reminder just how much impact chemicals can also have on our loved pets.

Plants

I have read there are some plants that help to purify the air and many are listed on the internet.

Replacing Furniture and Sofas

I know a lot of people buy second-hand furniture or keep their old furniture to avoid new smells or fumes coming into their home. I have done both and was in need of another sofa because the sponging in mine was very worn. I only had a limited selection of new sofas because I thought about buying one off a showroom floor but was worried about people who may have sat on it and left different smells on the fabric and what timbers were used to make it.

I had an idea, why not just replace all the sponging in my old sofa and problem solved. I checked with the upholsterer to ensure the sponge didn't have formaldehyde in it and it all worked out fantastic and cheaper.

I also put a throw rug over my sofa and arm chair, to protect it from any smells, then I can easily wash it and it stops smells going onto the fabric of my sofa.

Sweeping and Mopping

As previously mentioned, I purposely built my home with highly polished concrete floors throughout and no carpet anywhere which has been great for cleaning. When cleaning skirting's and bench tops, a long-handled stick microfiber wand is used as the dust sticks to it. My floors are dry microfiber mopped to collect dust and it limits dust fluffing up. Next, they are sprayed and mopped with another microfiber mop and a non-chemical eucalyptus-based product that leaves every room smelling fresh and clean. It's taken me years to work through different products to find one that work for me.

CHALLENGING PLACES, PRODUCTS or ACTIVITIES

Since moving out of suburbia and closer to the beach to enjoy the sea air, I have less bad air days. Also having my Plan of Action and Air Detective skills, I try to head out and not lock myself away so much. Sometimes my RADS will still catch me by surprise and I'll end up having breathing issues and sore lungs, however using my Plan of Action has kept me out of hospital and that's a very good thing! So, when I am having a "good air day" I will continue to try new things.

.

Appointments – Doctor & Specialist

My doctors and specialist post RADS have all been great. If there have been any renovations or painting at their surgery, then they call to let me know and move my appointments.

Once I arrive, if the waiting room has a number of people, I usually let the reception staff know that I am waiting outside in my van to avoid scented products. My doctor will usually wave to me when it's time to come in or their staff will call me on my phone when it's my time. I really appreciate staff doing this for me.

I have also been able to Skype with my specialist and psychologist to save me having to drive to the city and avoid all the fumes and potential breathing issues. This has been a huge help and greatly appreciated.

Appointments and treatment – Dentist

I am sad to say that trying to find a Dentist who would accommodate my sensitivities has been an ongoing and difficult task. Soon after I was diagnosed with RADS I had to see a Dentist as my front tooth had completely cracked. I eventually found a lovely Dentist who went out of her way to accommodate me. Sadly, only being new with RADS I didn't have my Plan of Action and wasn't able to provide her with any direction, nor was I aware of how reactive I was going to be to a common dental product called bond. As soon as she put the bond on my tooth, I had a severe reaction as the fume blew down my throat and my airways snapped shut and I began to suffocate. It was a very frightening and traumatic situation and the Dentist acted swiftly and grabbed two suction hoses and sucked the smell out of my mouth and kept doing it as I was gasping for air. I believe her swift action saved my life. Eventually my airways settled and I was able to breathe and gargle and spit out clean water to help further dissipate the trigger.

That was a difficult and scary lesson for me to learn and now years later I have had to have further dental work done and since moving it's still been hard to find a Dentist who would see me. Eventually I found one who has been wonderful and that's great!

I have made up a list below of information that may be useful to you and your Dentist that I have learnt over the years:-

- Find a dentist / dental surgeon who is willing to accommodate your RADS.
- I try to always book to be the first appointment of the day – limits exposure to others.
- I sometimes sit out in my car and the receptionist will phone me to come inside when ready.
- Explain your known sensitivities.
- Create a PLAN with your Dentist in regard to what happens IF you have a reaction as I did. Explained below:-
  When testing a product that is new to me – my dentist now tests it AWAY from me i.e. not put it under my nose to see if I have a reaction. They open the product at the door and slowly bring it toward me and if I am sensitive to it, I will usually have an immediate reaction (i.e. voice changes, begin to cough etc.) before they are too close. Then we know I cannot use it and I use oxygen from my small tank to blow the smell away from me while my airways slowly calm back down.
- I have normal water for gargling – i.e. no mouth wash products etc.
- Asking your Dentists and assistants to please not wear fragrances/lotions/scented soaps etc. when they see or operate on you.
- I call one day before to remind the Dentist and assistance about zero fragrance/scented products.
- If a Dentist or assistant has strong hair product (i.e. they forgot I was coming) My Dentist has wrapped their hair in a towel to smother the smell while doing a procedure on me – I find the flimsy hair nets do not contain the smell of strong hair conditioners and the smell seeps out.
- Non latex is used.
- Sterilizing units are put in a separate room away from me.
- Low adrenalin is used when I need an injection.
- Prepare to possibly pay a little more.

Not being able to have bond used on my teeth has made it a real challenge for my dentists working on my teeth and I have opted for those cracking to be extracted. Strangely I lost 5 teeth in one year?

Appointments and treatment – Denture / Partial Plates

At this time, I have had to get a partial denture plate made and as luck would have it, I found a great denture technician who does his best to limit any chemicals in his rooms. I now know the following about my reactions and what has helped me:-

- Having a separate laboratory from his surgery (limits my exposure to chemicals).
- To make the impressions he used a product called Alginate from Cavex Impressional made in Holland and I did not have any reaction.
- My plate is made MMA free and although it is a tiny bit smelly it's not causing me any breathing issues.
- Unfortunately, I had a fast and strong reaction to the tissue conditioner they used. It was put on my plate and I had the plate in my mouth for too long (about 15 minutes thinking the taste would dissipate... it didn't and my breathing got worse and worse. It took me about five days to get the taste out my mouth and system)
- I also had a strong reaction to a clear product that was supposed to be the same product as my current MMA plate. All we can put it down to was a bad batch. It took five days for the taste to leave my mouth and my system, with a lot of gargling. It has since been cleaned off and the pink MMA free product has been used again, with success.

BBQ

I was recently at a friend's home and she cooked a BBQ. I tried to sit outside but that only lasted a few seconds due to the cooking smells and smoke from the BBQ.

My solution was, I went inside away from any BBQ odour and chatted through the closed glass doors until the cooking was done and then I went back outside once the smell had dissipated. I am pleased to say that worked. If I go to another BBQ, I will arrange ahead of time to offer to make the salad inside while the BBQ is being cooked.

Built Up Area's and Cities

The pollution in the city, smog and fumes from cars and trucks in built up areas is extremely bad for my RADS and has caused me serious breathing issues.

My solution is, where possible I stay home and use Skype or other programs for face to face appointments rather than having to go into the city or built up areas. If I absolutely have to go to the city, then I either drive up on the weekend (less traffic) and stay in my van somewhere safe or I drive up the night before once all the traffic has settled down. I stay in my van somewhere safe overnight and go to my appointment the next day. I can't tell you how frustrating it was during my litigation that I had to attend numerous appointments in the city and even with all the strategies I did to reduce the impact on my health, I would still end up spending days or weeks to get over the exposures.

When I am travelling, I try to avoid driving through cities or built up areas that may have pollution and high traffic so I drive around, under or over the top, even if it adds miles to my trip.

Naturally I would have all the items listed under my RADS Tool Kit with me to assist if I am faced with a trigger and having my Plan of Action means I have the tools to manage any breathing issues I may have.

Camping / Caravan Parks

Campfires near me are a danger and my van allows me to pack up quickly and get away. Whatever other hazards that affect my breathing, my van allows me to move away.

It's important to be mindful of dust as it can be stirred up when people drive in and out of campsites and the smell of smoke and gas from cooking outside on portable stoves. Once I was designated a spot next to cigarette smoker and had to close my roof hatch and go into lock down due to the smell wafting into my van and causing me serious breathing issues.

Some caravan sites have laundry rooms and they are usually near the amenity's facility and bathrooms, which is challenging for me as many laundries in parks I have stayed in, have detergent smells wafting out of them.

I find the smell of damp earth and damp leaves can cause me breathing issues and if I am near a stream or water, I need to be mindful of mould spores.

My solution has been to park at showgrounds or free camp sites where you are not squeezed next to other campers and there is usually some space between your van and other travelers. I usually try to get up early and be the first person to use the shower which minimizes my exposure to scented products. If you can park at a site that has lawn to park on instead of dirt it usually limits the amount of dust going into your van/camp.

I have my CB Radio to call for help if I am in a non-mobile range and if I am doing long trips, I make sure someone knows what my travel plans are, where I am heading and I try to stay in touch each day. My preference is to travel near the coast because my airways and lungs always feel better near the ocean air and I avoid inland as much as possible, however living in Australia it can be difficult.

Also, I have "alert apps" on my phone which let me know about any bushfires, floods or storms and any pending controlled burn-offs.

I make sure I have a full large tank of medical air and 2 x full small tanks of oxygen and plan my trip knowing where I can get refill tanks.

I check what time of year I am travelling and avoid places where there maybe bush fires or farmers burning off. There are some great websites that will show last year's weather and future forecasts, so they can be really helpful when planning a trip away.

Also checking what the temperature and climate will be like is also very important.

Caves – Sightseeing

On my travels over to Western Australia I thought I would stop and check out the caves and the fact you enter at ground level, I thought I would be ok.

Soon after walking in I noticed the air was cold and I could smell and taste minerals. I tried to keep walking slowly and took some photos but could feel my airways restricting, so I turned around and made my way back outside to clean air. I began coughing once I was out and after a few minutes I could feel a chill in my lung, so I rested laying in my van at the beach and eventually the chill and pain in my lung subsided. At this time, no cave sightseeing for me. *(below is the quick photo I took inside the Mammouth Caves in WA)*

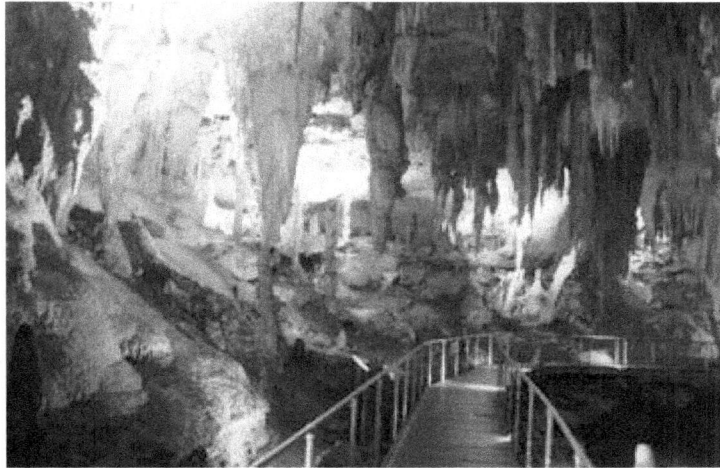

Cinema / Movie Theatre

I have had to leave the movies due to the smell from someone sitting a few rows behind me, after they sprayed aftershave or perfume that filtered down to me and immediately affected my breathing.

My solution is when possible, I sit at the very back so no-one can sit behind me and well away from others. I usually go to the movies in the day time when there are less people and not in school holidays.

I take my hand fan, water bottle and empty one, my P2 mask for the bathroom and I usually take my small oxygen tank with me. If however I am parked right out the front and I am having a good air day and there are not many people inside, I may leave my tank in the van.

Dancing

I used to love to go dancing and meet up with friends pre RADS and then after I was injured and I tried to go, I only lasted a short time and had serious breathing issues, either from perfume, cigarette smoke or if they had one of those smoke/fog machines running. It could have me sick for days or weeks depending on the trigger. I remember feeling pretty depressed about it and stayed away for a long time however once I created my Plan of Action, I found a new smaller dance place and I tried going and I did ok for a short time. So that lifted my spirits and motivated me to get dressed up and head out now and then.

I soon realized if I went in a little later the smell of perfume and aftershave wasn't so strong and I would try to place myself near a door or window and hope I could get some fresh air. Once I stood right under the air-conditioner and lasted a good while but it was pretty darn cold.

Nowadays, my preference is to go out to dinner and have a nice meal with great company. If there is an opportunity to go to a place for a dance, I wouldn't say no. At this point in my life, it's more about how tired I am and if my feet are sore and less worry about my breathing, which is great because .. you got it .. I have my Plan of Action. ☺

Gyms

I have tried going into eight different gyms with no luck. I found issues with the rubber smell from the actual gym equipment, carpet flooring, rubber mats, deodorants and other scented products. Many gyms had installed automatic chemical/fragrant sprays which waft around the gym and in the bathrooms to try to mask body odor and they caused me immediate breathing difficulties. One may need to be aware of the wipe downs some gyms use on the equipment as they could contain chemical products.

My solution was to create my own little gym at home. I recognize the importance of exercise for my health and wellbeing. Using my gym consistently is the part I need to improve on!

Hardware Stores

I used to enjoy going to have a wander through our large local hardware store however since getting RADS I have to wear my heavy-duty mask and I usually get in and out quite fast. This is mostly due to the smell of dust throughout the store/warehouse. I try to avoid the paint section as the smells can be quite strong and I keep well away from the wood section and potting mix area as they are usually disastrous for me. A strong smell of petrol can sometimes be found at the counter where you pay because that's where some hired tools are dropped off, so if I detect any smell of petrol, I don't bother going into the store, instead I leave and make a plan to go back another day.

The staff have generally been helpful getting items for me down isles that are just too smelly and difficult for me to go down. I try to do my research online first and find what I need and sometimes I will call the store and they will have the item waiting for me at the counter. That's wonderful when it happens and there's no petrol items on the counter before I get there.

Hair Dressers

Due to ammonia, conditioning treatments and other smells usually omitting from hairdressing salons that can cause me breathing issues, I usually avoid them. I did find a hairdresser who worked from home and she did my hair outside on her back porch. This worked well however washing out the hair dye in her laundry sink was extremely challenging. I would have my oxygen mask on but still end up inhaling some fumes from the product she used and that resulted in very sore lungs. So, I stopped going and did it myself in my backyard, using my masks and medical air as needed.

As previously mentioned, I built an outside shower at my home so I could wash products or dye out of my hair and not contaminate the inside of my home. As also mentioned, I have now found a hairdressing salon that does not have any products with chemicals, so I am thrilled and hope it's the way of the future not only for those of us with sensitivities but also for the many people working in salons.

Hospitals

I believe some hospitals have a policy for accommodating people who have MCS (Multiple Chemical Sensitivities) however others may not. In my experience I have been to hospitals that did not have this policy in place and was often left in the general waiting room where I have been exposed to people coming in wearing fragrances and exposed to hospital staff wearing fragrance, causing me further breathing issues. One hospital tried to separate me from other waiting patients by putting me in the children's waiting room however that became a problem when the mothers came in because one of them was wearing a strong fragrance and I had to immediately leave. I was then put in a corridor down the end of a hallway to wait, which was fine because no-one came near me.

My solution is, the last time I went to hospital, I explained what RADS was and asked to be put in an isolated room with no people and that medical air helps to settle my airways and my breathing. The hospital found the medical air outlet in the heart recovery department and put me in there with no-one else and I was able to use an old tube to breathe the medical air and it helped to relax my airways and settle my breathing. A nurse who didn't wear any fragrance regularly checked on me and once my breathing had settled and I was feeling ok, I was cleared to go home.

Now having a medical air tank at home and oxygen tank in my car has eliminated the need for me to go to hospital for my breathing issues. Yay!

Hotels

In hotels I have learnt to be very aware of smells the minute I walk in. At one there was a very strong "deodorizer" smell as I walked in. I spoke to the Manager and she confirmed that's what it was and that it filtered through the air-conditioning unit, so I had to leave as it was too overwhelming.

Some older hotels can have such a strong beer smell engrained into the carpet and it's just too strong for me to stay. Another hotel had a wonderful big open wood fire going but the smoke fumes were an issue, so I had to leave.

At many hotels I notice staff using a pink or blue substance in spray bottles to wipe down tables or benches. I can smell it at 100 paces and no-one seems to know what is in it. I just know it gives me severe breathing issues if the smell comes my way, so I hate to think what impact it has on those using it. I will usually try to chat to the staff about how important it is to protect their lungs and if they have to use those pink or blue cleaning products, then at least just spray it into a cloth and then wipe the table and maybe hold their breath so they don't breathe it in.

Although I have had a myriad of different breathing experiences calling into some hotels, when I am away travelling, I will continue to pop into some, as it's nice to meet locals and support small town business. I just have to play it by ear and rely on my Plan of Action if I have an issue.

Hot Springs

There are gorgeous hot springs not too far from where I used to live, so I decided to go as it had lots of different outdoor pools and spas and thought I would be ok. I lasted a little while in an outside hot spring spa that was situated on the top of a hill with a great breeze blowing. Once the breeze stopped though I had to get out because the heat mixed with the minerals and steam caused me to have breathing issues.

Regrettably, I had to leave the resort and it took me over a week to recover as I ended up with severe pain in my lungs.

My solution at this stage, is to give them a miss. Although one day in the future I may try another one on the other side of town as I had a conversation with another RADS Warrior who had been there and didn't experience any breathing or lung issues. So that was encouraging.

Laundromats

I try to avoid walking past laundromats because of the smell of laundry powder and fabric softener that can filter out. Only on a couple of occasions, when I have been away did I need to use them and lucky for me, one had a huge front door that stayed wide open allowing the smell of the various detergents to filter out. The second one, the door was closed, so I put my mask on and held my breath while I put a load in and then waited outside in my van for it to finish.

My solution has been, when I am away to wash out my underwear each night. If I have to use a laundromat, I always make up my own washing liquid before going in, so it's less time to be inside the laundromat and I wear my mask and hold my breath.

It's a bit of a lottery if your clothes are going to come out smelling of a previously used detergent after being in a commercial machine. I must be lucky because so far so good!

If you have a partner or friend who can go to the laundromat for you and use your detergent solution, this would be helpful.

I try to take a week of clothes when I am away to avoid having to use laundromat. Mind you there is a new laundromat that has recently opened in our little shopping complex and I must say I very tentatively stepped inside to say hello to a friend and I was able to breathe ok. So, it can be hit or miss.

Library

The library's I have gone into have been very challenging and I think it's due to all the books with all those paper fibers, fine dust and usually it's their carpet too. I also have problems being near all the newspapers that are usually on display at our local library when you walk in. The ink seems to be an especially strong trigger for me, so knowing this I hold my breath to get past them and I don't stay in the library long.

My solution is to check online first to see if they have the book or DVD etc. I want and ask if they can have it at the counter waiting for me. They are always helpful and obliging and it limits the time I am in there.

Lifts

I have done very cautious sniff tests before stepping inside lifts and when they have been too smelly to go in, I would need time to get over having sniffed something that I reacted to. It's situations like this that are so frustrating for people who have RADS. We can't control who might get into the lift prior or with us and we never know if they are wearing perfume, aftershave, body lotion, hair spray etc. and how severely we may react to it. It's all very unpredictable!

If a person has worn a fragrance in a lift it can sometimes take a while for the smell to dissipate, so I either use the stairs if it's not far, however they can harbor fumes or use another lift or try to wait it out. That's as long as my sniff test hasn't caused me serious enough issues that I have to leave.

On the other hand, the lift may be ok, however you won't know until you are there and I have learnt to always be prepared due to the fact it's such a small confined space. If I knew I was going to an appointment where I may have to use a lift then I would take my small oxygen tank, hand fan, mask and bottle of water. I would let the people at the appointment know ahead of time about the potential of me not being able to use the lift and possibly being late or having to cancel.

My solution was to start requesting the appointment be via internet meeting programs instead of placing myself in a high-risk situation. Some people and companies were able to accommodate this, so I was grateful and very glad I asked.

Motels

Most of the motels I have tried to stay in have caused me breathing issues due to the chemicals used to clean the room and the detergent used to wash the sheets and towels or some other anomaly. I also had issue with the roof at one place because it was made of straw and I only lasted a short time before having to leave due to the fine dust falling down and the smell of the straw. At another motel the housemaid swished water and bleach on all the pathways outside the motel doors, so I stayed inside with my air purifier running flat out.

My solution was to always have my air purifier with me and my own bedding. At some places I would take all the blankets off the bed and smother the carpet with them as some motels would sprinkle deodorizer over the carpet. Calling ahead is a good idea and speaking with Management and letting them know you have sensitivities and ask if they could take products out that have fragrances or scents, like room deodorizers, soaps etc. Another alternative would be to open all doors and windows and use something like pegs or a tie to pull back curtains to air the room on arrival and put the air-conditioned on.

Since having my campervan, I rarely need to stay in motels anymore, which has reduced my exposure to the above.

Nail Technician

If I see a nail shop that is on my path while out shopping, I usually hold my breath when I pass by or I walk to the other side of the path due to the strong fumes they can omit.

Office and Buildings

For me, walking into any building or office with RADS can be a mine-field of triggers or it could be ok. Based on what has happened to me in the past, my Air Detective skills ramp up in this environment because it can be so unpredictable.

There are so many factors to take into account like:- the air quality in the office or building, when were the floors last mopped and what with, when was reception last cleaned and with what, how dusty is the floor, is there carpet, how long ago were the carpets vacuumed, are air "fresheners" used or diffusers at the reception desk, has anyone just walked through with a strong aftershave or perfume, are there any newspapers in the waiting room, are there any open windows and if so which way are they facing and will traffic fumes blow in etc.

I have had to leave various appointments due to different triggers that have caused me breathing issues. I left an appointment due to the smell of the ink and the new paper from freshly printed reports that had been placed on the counter top of the reception where I was standing. I immediately left another appointment after a person walked into the reception area and stood next to me with a "deep heat" type antiseptic smell on their arm and in one breath I had immediate breathing difficulties.

On another occasion I didn't even last a minute in a building after walking into the reception area that had a very strong smell coming from the carpet. It wasn't a deodorizer smell, more so a mould smell from water damage.

I walked out of another building due to the extremely strong perfume the reception staff were wearing.

My solution, where possible I use Skype or speak via teleconference software from home and eliminate having to go into buildings or offices for appointments. If it's unavoidable I will usually call ahead and explain I have RADS and ask a few questions just to limit the potential of a trigger. I always have my small oxygen tank, water and masks with me and having my Disability Tag on my van means I can usually park close by in the event I have to exit the building fast, unless in the city where there is very limited parking.

Outdoor Events

I went along to a local music festival thinking it would be ok because it was on a large lawn area but it was set up in a circle. The food vans were very close together and there were heaps of people in the middle. The cooking smells and the smells from the crowd were trapped in the middle and were not being blown away. This triggered my breathing issues and I had to leave.

I tried to go to an outdoor market in front of the beach up on the lawn but the layout had all the tents in a row opposite each other and people walked down the middle like a long snake. The perfume from people and smells from stalls was too strong being wafted down the middle of the snake like path, so I had to leave.

My solution is to keep trying but not to place myself in harm's way. I did see it was going to be a windy day at the beach when the markets were next on so I went along and it was great that time, as the wind blew most of the smells away.

On one of my travels, I went to another outdoor market and it was around a huge oval with lots of gentle breeze which blew away fumes from the food vans and scented candle stalls etc., so I was able to walk around and enjoy all the colorful items being sold. They are a lot of fun and it was great to be out and about.

I would love to go to an outdoor concert again as I did prior to getting RADS so that's a new plan I will have to create and I am hopeful it will happen!

My above experiences highlight the importance of a clean breeze and hopefully it's blowing in the right direction and not blowing fumes toward me. I've become quite good at maneuvering myself to be in the best optimal position to take in good clean air and quickly dodge people or hold my breath if I get any hint of an odor to minimize my exposure.

Ozone Machine

In an effort to try to sleep in my bedroom and remove whatever smell/ chemical is causing me breathing issues, I did some research and read that an Ozone Machine might help to remove some odors. So, after asking questions to a local company I hired one. They suggested I run the machine in the closed room for about 8 hours. Fortunately, I removed my clothes from the room and put a large sheet over my bed and had towels pushed up by the door which kept the horrendous smell in the one room.

This was sadly a total disaster for me!

Upon re-entering the room to turn off the machine I had to wear two masks, and put a folded towel hard up to my face, hold my breath and run in and turn off the machine and quickly open the windows and sliding door. Upon leaving the room, the ozone smell (which some seeped through the masks and towels, smelt to me like very strong chlorine) was all over my clothes, in my hair and on my skin and I had to quickly strip off and shower and wash my clothes. I was told by the company it should dissipate after about two to three days. Even keeping my windows and sliding door open, I was not able to walk back into that room for many weeks without having a breathing issue.

My solution is that sometimes methods or items I try go wrong or don't work for my personal situation. This incident is a reminder to test a small area first whenever possible.

Parking

When I am heading to the beach, I am very mindful of which way the wind is blowing and where I park my van. If I am sitting in my van on what I call "good air days" I have to ensure I park right next to the ocean and not across the road because I get the fumes of passing cars blowing toward my van. When I am parked in a great position getting lovely clean air, sometimes people walk past and the breeze can blow their perfume, sunscreen or insect repellent through my open window or open sliding door and into my van causing me breathing issues.

I don't park in any closed underground car parks for the obvious reason of fumes lingering, which means it's a potential RADS disaster for me. The city can have very limited parking, so I would park just out of the city and get a taxi in. (which can present a whole other set of problems)

As previously mentioned, having a Disability Tag has been an enormous help to me in providing parking spots that generally have good access to entry and front doors, which limits my exposure to fumes and triggers.

Pharmacy / Chemist

It seems many chemists now sell washing powder, perfume, diffusers and a collection of other scented products inside the store and on display out the front. This can make it very challenging just getting through the door!

If I do have to venture in, I wear my mask and have learnt to hold my breath as well. I work out a master plan to dodge all the various fumes and get to the back where the prescription counter is without contaminating myself.

I did recently learn that I can actually leave my script there and call ahead for repeats and they can get my medication ready for me, so that's great and saves me waiting around, instead I just walk in and pick it up.

For days when I am not well, I am also aware that some chemists offer a home delivery service, so then you don't even have to leave home, which sounds really helpful.

Public Bathrooms and Showers

Many of those air scented products that automatically spray out smells in bathrooms are a major issue for me as well as many of the cleaning chemicals. I walked up to a bathroom that had been sprayed with bleach and hosed down, so I didn't even make it to the door before having to immediately leave and head for my oxygen. When travelling on the road here in Australia there are some toilets on the side of the roads where there are truck stops and pull overs to rest between towns and some have toilets called a "long drop." Basically, they are a toilet seat that is set over a long hole in the ground and if you lift up the lid to sit on the toilet, then you get all the sewerage fumes from below which can be overwhelming and cause me severe breathing issues. Consequently, I avoid these toilets at all costs.

In emergency bathroom situations, I will use a toilet in a hotel or fast-food place and I am very good at holding my breath and staying calm!

My solution is I mostly use the Disability bathroom as they are larger and don't seem to hold as many strong smells from perfume products. In a small place like a bathroom, if there is a "line up" of people waiting this can be very challenging with people standing very close to me wearing scented products.

Some public bathrooms stink of urine and this is a trigger, so I would use my P2 mask and try to hold my breath for as long as I can. Having my van with a little portable loo has been great for those quickie bathroom stops where I can be safe in my van, no people and no chemicals. Eventually I would love to get a van that has a shower and this would mean I don't have to find or use public showers or showers in caravan parks when I am away travelling.

Public showers can be a haven for scented products and also because the fragrance can linger long after people have left.

My solution for showering when I am away is, I try to get up very early and be the first person in and out the shower area. When I am away in my van and if there are no showers I have done the following:- I fill up two large plastic two liter empty bottles with water. Put the lid on them and rest them on the dash of my van, so they get nice and warm. I have sewn three shower curtains together so they wrap around my back-van doors when they are open. I use a spare lid that fits the bottles of water and punch little holes in it with a nail and put it on one of the bottles of warm water. I then stand in a big bucket behind the curtains at the back of my van and grab the bottle with the lid that has holes in it and squirt the warm water over me and have a quick shower under the stars. Sounds primitive but it works.

Thanks to my Uncle Graham for creating that solution. ☺ (I'm still going to save for a van with a shower in it though!)

Restaurants

At one restaurant I explained that I could not eat any pepper but sadly one pepper corn snuck into my meal and when I bit on it, I had an abrupt and severe breathing issue where I began to suffocate. I immediately put my Plan of Action into place and fortunately paramedics were not needed due to having my oxygen tank in my van nearby. I sipped on water and although I was coughing a lot, I remained calm and waved the oxygen tube near my mouth and eventually my airways settled and my coughing stopped. Fortunately, my friend with me was left to explain to the waiter what was happening and why I fled the restaurant. We drove to the beach and sat on a bench taking in the sea breeze until I felt well enough to leave.

I will try to go to different restaurants so that I can figure out which ones are good for me and those that aren't. If one seems ok, then I will usually go and check the bathroom to test if it's ok for me to be in as well. If it has strong scents spraying automatically then I will either leave or make a note to go to the bathroom before going to the restaurant.

Some restaurants have open kitchens and sometimes the smells coming from the kitchen are too overwhelming for me, so I don't stay. Others have had a fire burning for ambiance or a large pizza oven and the smell of wood smoke is so bad for my RADS that I walk in and then out.

Some restaurants pack people in very tight, so they are sitting very close to me so I usually avoid these places.

My solution for going into a restaurant does depend on many things and generally I have noticed I am usually good if the venue has good airflow, room between the tables, if it's a larger room and the bathrooms don't smell of fragrance or strong cleaning chemicals. If all is ok, then I will book early and get a table near the back and away from people (if possible) and while I used to be in and out before more people arrive, I have been pushing that boundary lately and so far, so good!

I have found the best restaurants for my RADS are those at or on the beach where there is an outside eating area. I usually try to get a table where there is a sea breeze blowing toward me. A lot of outside dining can be near a road and that usually means traffic and fumes, in those situations I will sit inside to eliminate this.

I try to get out to a restaurant a couple of times a month and it's wonderful even though sometimes things don't always work out. Having been cooped up inside for so long and isolated, it's so nice just being out and socializing, so when it all works out, it's great! If I happen to have a waiter or waitress who is wearing a strong fragrance, I will do whatever I need to dissipate the trigger. Once I am ok to speak, I have a polite conversation with the Manager and explain I am reacting to the staff members fragrance and in these few cases, they have been extremely understanding, allocating a different staff member to wait on our table.

Smells and Tastes

I cannot be around incense, sparklers, lit matches (sulphur is especially bad), scented candles, burning candles, lavender, tea tree oil and other oils. I have found that the taste or smell of pepper, chili, garlic or cinnamon can also give me breathing issues of different levels.

Receiving gifts of flowers can be problematic because some fresh cut flowers can give me breathing issues and I don't know which ones until I am in smelling range.

A few more triggers are cigarette smoke, wood smoke, many spray deodorants, perfumes, aftershave, body washes, lotions, scented soaps, nail polish, diesel fumes, petrol fumes, motor oils, fabric softeners, gas, pesticides, bark, paint, air fresheners, washing detergents, numerous cleaning products, VOC's, new rubber, new plastic, chlorine, mould, formaldehyde, fire retardants on clothes, block out on curtains, fresh ink, paper fiber, sulphur, some felt pens, dog dander, dust, some cooking oils, some cooking smells and timber just to name a few.

Even the strong smell of rubbish in the bin can cause me to have a reaction, so I've become good at holding my breath when doing particular jobs and I usually wipe my empty bin with a tiny bit of eucalyptus so it smells nice and fresh.

My solution is now that I have such an acute sense of smell and my Air Detective skills are in good form, I can usually divert or move away from a fume or pollutant smell before inhaling too much, all reducing the negative impact on my health.

Listening to my body is very important, as well as staying calm and no longer having drama and/or anxiety latching on is great.

As mentioned previously, I carry a water bottle and a smaller empty bottle so if I do come into contact with a smell or fume and I can taste it I n my mouth, then I simply gargle and spit it out a few times and I have found this really helps me. Prior to rinsing out my mouth, I would wake up the next day and I could taste whatever I had breathed in the previous day in my throat and in my saliva. It was terrible but since gargling and spitting this has reduced.

Prior to being diagnosed with RADS, one medical professional suggested when I knew I was going out to the shops, to put Vaseline in my nose to block any smells and just breathe through my mouth. This proved disastrous for me because a lady close by was wearing perfume and I could not smell it but I could taste it and my airways immediately began to restrict and I began suffocating. This taught me an important lesson as to how very important my sense of smell is. I need my nose to be free of any smell or product like Vaseline to allow my Chief Air Assessor to do his job and smell and assess the air I breathe and together we keep me safe!

Sparklers, Birthday Candles and Incense

My family bought me a birthday cake one year and as they brought it out, I saw it had a few sparklers pushed into the cake. I didn't think anything about it until they came closer and I had severe breathing issues due to the strong smell of sulphur the sparklers omitted and I had to leave the room and use my oxygen straight away to dissipate the fumes from my airways. I know I am the same with candles, smoke and if someone lights a match.

My solution is an easy fix, by not having any lit candles on any of my Birthday cakes in the future. Also, if I am at a place where there are Birthday candles or sparklers being lit, then I just leave the room until it's dissipated. Recently at my 60th Birthday my son and his partner surprised me with two amazing birthday cakes and they did something ingenious. They put battery operated flashing candles on my birthday cakes, so **no fumes** and no trouble with my breathing! The thought in that blew me away and I was really grateful.☺

I don't come into contact with incense often other than catching a little smell when avoiding the meditation shop and when I order Indian food at our local Indian restaurant. They have a large cupboard full of incense near their pay station, so they kindly close the doors on the cupboard when I go in to pay. I do appreciate it but it's still quite strong and I do my best to hold my breath and get in and out fast. Wish I didn't love their Butter Chicken so much!

Spas and Sauna

The places I have tried to walk into have either diffusers or scented candles burning and are filled with smells that trigger me. I just find it too overwhelming.

I did try using a sauna but the smell of the timber caused me breathing issues so I tried a different sauna that was not as bad until I stepped out and a lady walked past with some body lotion on that was very strong. Although my airways reacted to her fragrance, I knew what to do to help myself and followed my Plan of Action. At the end of the day I was still very pleased with myself that I tried.

My solution was, I saved up and included a spa bath in my plans when constructing my home so I could have a little indulgence. I also did some research on near infrared sauna lights which looked interesting.

Swimming Centers

If there is an outside pool, I am generally ok however the battle has been getting to it. Having to walk into an indoor Swimming Centre to get to the outside pool area has been too difficult due to very strong chlorine smells.

My solution has been to find an outside swimming pool that is saltwater chlorinated and not within a big complex. I did find one that is 30 minutes from my home, which has been worth the drive on very hot days.

If I had a partner, maybe they could pay and speak to the attendants at the counter of the large Swimming Centre while I walk past holding my breath. That could possibly work. Mind you, I would probably need to wash the smell of chlorine off my body in their showers and that could present other issues.

Tennis

Tennis can be a lot of fun, so I went along to a small social club and hoped the bushes would stop the fumes from the nearby main road but it didn't and I had breathing issues so I had to stop. I did try to play a social game at another court away from the road but the oval was right next to a new playground and the smell of new mulch and bark was too overwhelming for me.

My solution was to go in search of another court that was off the road and I found one. I also had the good fortune of meeting another person who doesn't wear scented products and they offered to have a gentle hit with me. So how good is that! Never give up!

ENVIRONMENT

I feel the environment plays a huge role in helping me live the best life I can with my RADS. In my opinion, to create a controlled environment that does not include any triggers, is easy to say but difficult to accomplish.

My RADS can be very unpredictable and so can the environment. Knowing I have my Plan of Action really helps to teach me to be calm when I'm presented with a trigger and get on with the job of minimizing my exposure. I no longer get stressed but rather plan ahead and manage situations as they present and log information that is useful.

Bays

There is a large bay about an hour or so from where I now live and large container ships and other sea vessels frequently go in and out. On certain days I could smell and taste pollution and fumes in the air, so it wasn't where I wanted to live. Prior to moving to the Surf Coast, I did random tests of the air quality over several years in different parts of the bay. Some areas were lovely and the air smelt quite clean, however for me the air at the Surf Coast had more ferocity when it was blowing in off the ocean and I could really taste the salt in the air, so that was the winner for me.

(Below is the beautiful Hardwicke Bay in South Australia)

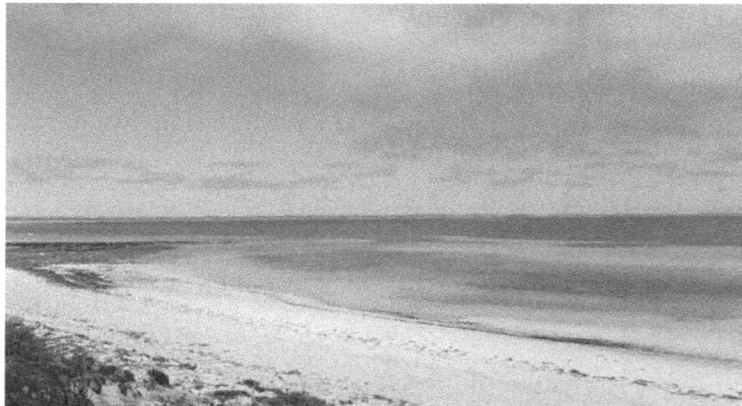

Dust

At this stage of reading my book, and the fact I have mentioned dust more than seventy times, I expect you already know that dust is another serious trigger for me.

If travelling, I usually plan my journey following a coastline to avoid it. As previously mentioned, I will keep my windows up, the air-conditioning on recycle. I also keep my throat saturated to avoid dust impacting on my airways.

In my video on YouTube®, RADS Awareness Trip Across Australia Part 2, you see firsthand the situations I am faced with when I did travel inland, so I take precautions to stay safe. Why did you do it, you may ask? Well it was to see relatives and to call into more hospitals to drop off flyers about RADS.

At home dust is my arch enemy, as I notice even the finest of dust can cause me various levels of breathing difficulties and being in a new housing area, it's an ongoing battle to minimize it coming into my home. This is also why I am very careful about *how* my home is cleaned, to minimize fluffing up dust.

I don't need much exposure to dust to have a reaction. It feels like fine powder has been sprinkled down my throat and onto my airway drying it out and causing immediate and at times, serious breathing issues. Within a short time, my lung usually becomes impacted and it feels very restricted, reducing how much oxygen I can breathe in, as well as experiencing pain with each breath.

So, I have learnt to remain calm, slow everything down, drink lots of water and immediately follow my Plan of Action.

Once I'm in a dust free environment, I need to be patient because it can take quite some time for my lungs to recover.

No doubt my solution is to avoid or reduce dust as best I can, where ever I am. Wearing my masks, having curtains to catch dust in my home and van, I've removed carpet and have my floors regular cleaned, which all helps.

Forest

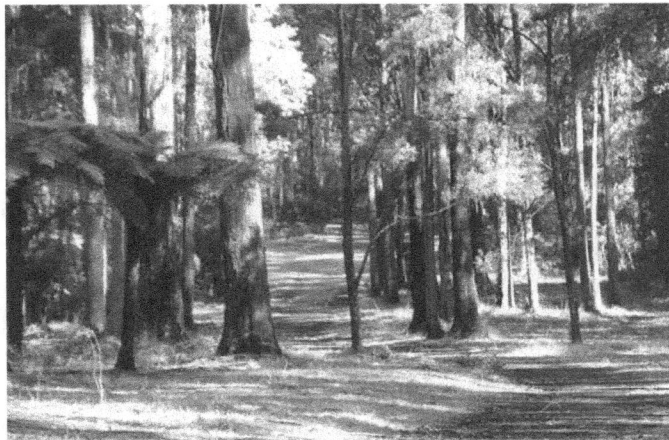

When I was at the beginning of my journey living with RADS, every day I was learning about my triggers and I found myself driving up to the forest desperate for relief of the severe breathing issues I was having. I spent months sitting in my car in the forest, breathing in the clean air that would eventually settle my airways.

I would try going for walks but realized I was not able to walk in all areas of the forest and noticed I was extremely reactive down near the streams where the air felt dense and humid. The smell of dampness in the soil on some of the walking tracks had my airways reacting.

My solution was to walk on dry tracks that were open to the sun and on concrete paths and when I did this, I didn't have any breathing issues.

Sometimes I would just lie on the back seat of my car with the window down and just breathe in the clean air. I always felt better after spending time in the forest.

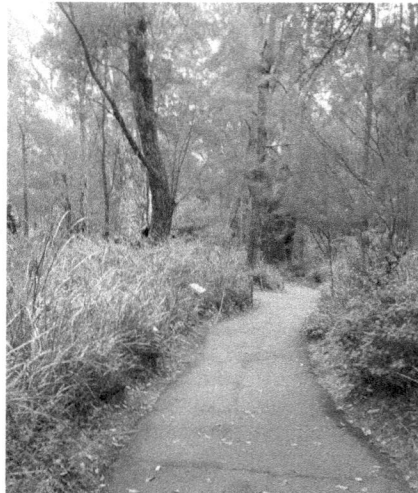

Humidity

Having only had limited exposure to humidity since having RADS, when interstate friends told me how much they enjoyed visiting a famous large zoo up north, I started to think about the prospect of going.

I did my research checking what time of year had the least humidity and thought I would give it a go. I packed everything from my RADS Tool Kit in my van and everything else, including way too many clothes (not unusual) and I took off feeling confident and well prepared.

It was a very long drive, (1,850km or 1,150 miles) and again, I was on my own. I was hoping I would cope with the humidity because after visiting the zoo,

I wanted to explore some of the amazing beaches and continue following the coastline.

Although I was still a couple of hours away from the zoo and I felt a little moisture in the air, I was doing ok! Great, so I continued and I kept the air-conditioner on in my campervan.

The higher up I travelled, the more humidity I experienced and although it was probably considered low humidity by locals, I was really surprised at how much it started to affect my breathing. I noticed my airways weren't reacting however my lung felt like it was becoming over saturated, like a heavy wet sponge, making my breathing feel laboured. Not a good feeling.

I made it to the zoo but just walking around was becoming a struggle. At one point I got onto a little train that was taking tourists to other parts of the zoo but sadly the fumes from that got trapped in the humid air and caused me even more issues. Oh, the joys of RADS! I had to take time out to rest and placed the oxygen tube from my small tank near my mouth to allow the moving oxygen to calm my airways. Fortunately, I had seen most of the zoo when this happened, so I decided the safe and sensible thing to do was, to leave. This was a good decision because it started to rain and the humidity was increasing.

So, I cut my trip short and drove back down south and within a couple of hours my breathing came back to normal. I felt much better and was so relieved to be breathing without any restriction.

I was proud of myself for achieving my goal of visiting to the zoo, however for now, I am simply going to avoid travelling where there is humidity.

Lakes

I have been to a few lakes in my travels since my injury and while many are lovely, I did miss the salt in the air. I have been to a couple of lakes where there were jet skis and ski boats and the smell of the petrol fumes carried across the water to where I was sitting. I moved but then the breeze changed and invaded my clean air. I ended up having breathing issues and left. Some lakes I have visited can be stagnant and smell, so I avoid staying too close to them.

My solution is, if I am going to stay at or near a lake, I check what type of activity there is on the lake and also check if there is a good breeze, which way the wind may be blowing and what is close by to the lake that may impact the clean air. *(Below is the picturesque Cockatoo Lake in South Australia)*

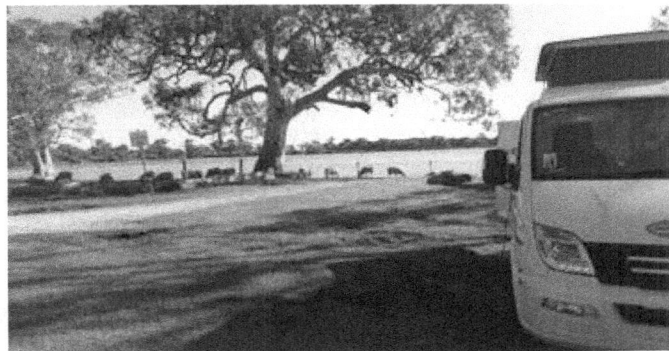

Ocean Air

Avoiding triggers and having my Plan of Action is a large factor in reducing my breathing issues and combining that with the healing and therapeutic benefits of breathing in clean salt air blowing in from the ocean, is a winning combination for me. Ocean air continues to heal the tenderness and pain in my lung after a strong exposure and calms my airways. Best of all, it's all natural!

So, after coming down here to the Surf Coast regularly to test my theory that the crashing waves creating negative ions and the amazing salt ocean air was so healing for me, I made the big decision to sell my home and move as close as I could to the ocean for my physical and mental health.

I know I'm not the only person with RADS who's had success with clean ocean air being such a game changer and it's why I promote it so much!

(Below is a photo I took at the amazing Bells Beach here at the Surf Coast)

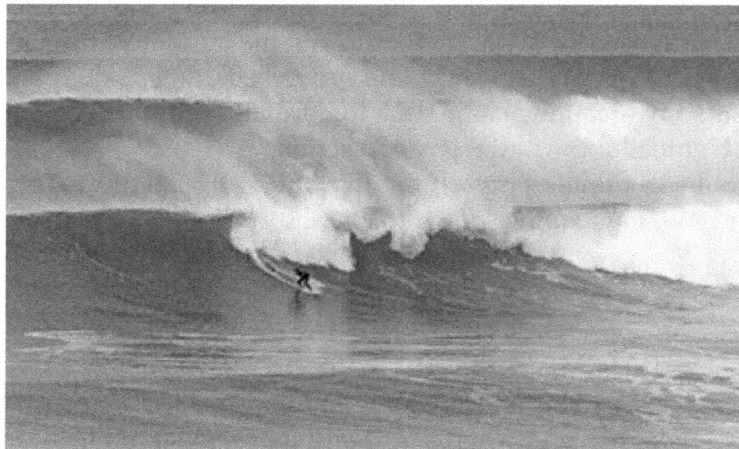

I understand that some RADS sufferers can live near a beach but still have issues with industry close by that blows pollution their way or they are in a humid climate. Finding a beach or ocean that has pristine air blowing in with no pollutants in a climate that suits your sensitivities can be a challenge. This took me some time searching to find and although I am still faced with some challenges like smoke or fumes blowing in from built up areas, I am grateful to have many good air days.

I was so desperate for the pain in my lungs to ease and/or the coughing to stop, I would make that long drive through traffic and past the city to get to where I now live. Sometimes I would get triggered on the trip down however once I began breathing in the ocean air, it eventually healed whatever breathing issues I had, and I felt so very good after. I would rest in my car with my window down to allow the healing salt air to blow in and with each breath the pain in my lung would slowly subside and my breathing would improve.

There were times I sat on the beach alone and cry just out of exhaustion and thankfulness that I could feel this good again. I had to keep this feeling in the forefront of my mind to motivate myself to keep making the long trip.

How many other people had to drive that far just so they could breathe without pain? It was ridiculous and sad all at the same time but I was so very glad to be there and to have found it.

This is why I made that big decision to sell my home in suburbia and move to this beautiful coastline beach.

I have spoken to others with RADS who have sold their homes and live fulltime in caravans or motorhomes following their coastline and just keep moving to chase the clean ocean air and good weather to limit triggers. I appreciate that's not practical or doable for everyone and that's why I purchased my van, so I can take off when the air here is being compromised or if I need to escape the cold in winter, or just for a change of scenery.

I appreciate there are many people with RADS who live inland, in cities or towns that are a very long way from any ocean or they are not in a position to travel that far. Maybe if you are able to find a compromise and head to a big lake, waterfall or a forest and enjoy the clean air.

I had no idea all those times I would leave my home and head off in different directions on a mission to find clean air that I would find myself down here along the Great Ocean Road. I am so fortunate and very grateful we have amazing beaches in Australia and wonderful ocean air. In my travels I have been to many beautiful beaches including those on the east coast of Australia, South Australia's coast and I travelled the south coast of Western Australia where the ocean air was wonderful.

I have learnt how important the wind is when I am planning to go to the beach because if it is blowing from the wrong direction then it may have pollution, dust or fumes so I won't go to the beach on those days.

Pollution

I learnt very early in my life living with RADS that pollution played a significant role in causing me severe breathing issues. Whether it was from built up cities, industrial areas or high traffic, I do my best to avoid it as much as I can. Even though I would have breathing issues at the time of inhalation of pollution, I would also suffer with the after effects of sensitive airways, lung inflammation and sometimes I would spit up blood the next day, (which has since been confirmed relates to my sinuses.) All this could take days or weeks to settle and heal, not to mention how frightening and painful it is.

Therefore, in an effort to avoid it, I try to go over or around built up areas and if I am able to, I would drive at night to reduce the impact of pollution. Nowadays, I also apply my mask and use my medical air if I cannot avoid a built-up area. Driving at night has been very successful for me in reducing or eliminating triggers, which is fantastic!

I am aware some people who live with RADS are very close to cities where they are faced with pollution every day and it's a big problem for them. To keep their homes as pollution free as possible they run air purifiers and make sure they wear good quality masks when going outside.

Smoke

Right now, as I sit here typing this, I am in my fourth day of being what I call "in lockdown" due to our beautiful town being engulfed with smoke blowing over from the devastating fires that are ravishing the east coast of Australia. *(Below is my local beach being invaded by smoke making it impossible for me to go for a walk)*

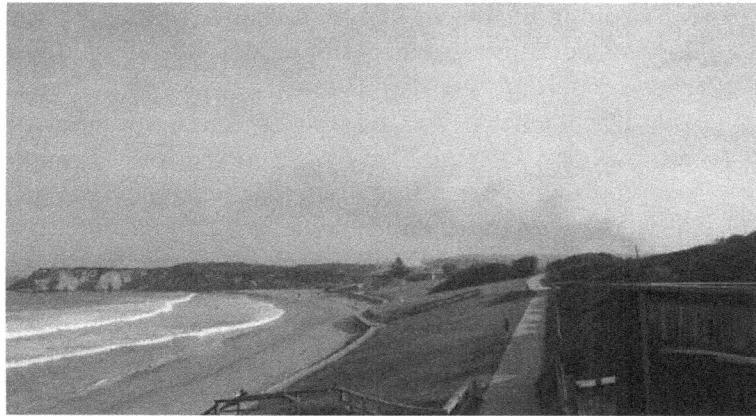

Living in Australia, I was brought up to respect the vast landscape and sadly fires are all too common here. When I designed my home, I did it with a deliberate focus on how I could keep smoke out in the event of a farmer's burn off or controlled burns. I am very happy to say that everything in my design for keeping smoke out of my home is working great as well as having air purifiers running, however I am going to need a few days out of my home to get over the lung pain I am experiencing from being inside my home for too long.

So back to smoke; Smoke can be a hazard to anyone's health and smoke for RADS sufferers is a very strong trigger and I do all I can to not be exposed to any.

There are many different masks on the market and while I'm yet to find one that offers 100% protection from smoke, there are a couple that come very close. When I have been in my vehicle and had to drive through smoke, not only do I wear my mask and have my medical air or oxygen tube placed under the chin, I also wet a face cloth and placed it over the nose of my mask to help limit exposure. It worked fine and I didn't have any serious breathing issues.

There are many great Apps (some are listed on our Facebook Group) that will provide warnings if there is smoke or a fire in my area and I am vigilant if I am going to be travelling, to check past weather reports and check when farmers do their burn offs etc. Doing your due diligence is important if you are going away or travelling.

If you have a neighbor who burns wood or has a flue pumping out smoke from a wood fire that can be a real issue and the only thing I have been able to do, to slow down its impact is close all my windows and doors, roll up towels and place them at the bottom of the doors and put some up against the base of window frames to stop smoke filtering in and pull my curtains shut. I also put on my extraction fans, as well as the extraction fan above the stove to help suck out any smoke. I run air purifiers and if I am still experiencing issues then I might leave and go to a large shopping complex that I know has good air-conditioning. I did recently go to a large supermarket that is very close by and wander around near the open fridge section where it's cold and has good air-conditioning. Within a short time, my breathing came good and I felt so much better, I just make sure I keep away from the other end of the supermarket where all the detergent isles are.

On some occasions when I think it's going to be a great air day, I might leave a window open and get caught out by coming home to some smell that's invaded my home. When this has happened, I turn on all my fans to blow the smell out and then lock up again. Fortunately, it doesn't happen very often. I would rather air my home than close everything. If I hear any reports of fires heading my way, then I immediately close all my windows and doors.

When building my home, I decided to build in a new area to avoid older homes that still burn wood in winter and produce a lot of smoke. I didn't count on the fire pits, which one of my neighbors lights up occasionally, thank goodness it's not often. To reduce the impact of smoke, as previously mentioned, I planted large shrubs as a buffer to filter the smoke and reduce it coming into my yard. If I have any clothes on the outside line, I would need to take them down so the smell of smoke isn't trapped in the fibers.

Then I have the hazard of dealing with cigarette smoke. I sometimes cross the road or hold my breath to avoid walking through or past smokers. Cigarette smoke lingers, much like perfume and scented products.

If I can see smoke or get one hint of smelling it, then I do the same thing I do with petrol fumes, perfume etc. and calmly hold my breath, then very slowly let the air out as I get away from it. If you have had smoke inhalation and your Plan of Action is not successful then go to hospital or call your local Emergency Number.

Summer – Extreme Heat

Extreme heat can also cause me to have labored breathing, so I do my best to avoid it.

My solution is to keep hydrated by drinking plenty of water and maybe go for a drive to find a place where there is a lovely sea breeze blowing off the ocean and hopefully there isn't a zillion tourists and cars.

(Below is my tent set up to catch some Vitamin D before the tourist invade)

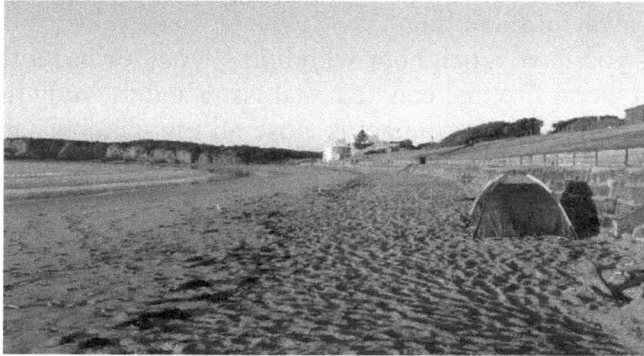

If I am at home, I will close all the curtains to reduce the heat coming into my home and I will have a few cool showers. If my floors have been recently damp mopped then I might put on some fans. I sometimes wipe the fan grate with peppermint or eucalyptus and then the air it blows out smells lovely and it's soothing on my lungs.

I've also been known to wander around the supermarket again, near the deli section where it's cold to just get some relief from the heat but don't tell anyone!

I have made provisions to install an air-conditioning unit in my home but at this stage I don't need one. I will definitely do some research before purchasing one to ensure it has a good hepa filter.

The Tasteless, Non-Smelling Trigger

Trust your body, listen to your body, feel how your breathing is feeling. That's the only way I have been able to detect what I call a "silent trigger" and it has only happened a couple of times since I have had RADS. Once when my home had been painted with a no VOC paint, I felt a reaction and impact on my airway and lung but my Air Detective skills were baffled and couldn't identify what the faint smell was. I removed myself and only spent limited time in my home off and on for about three years. During that time, I had other rooms repainted with different paint but still had the same physical reaction. It's nearly four years since my home was built and depending on my RADS and how reactive I am, I can usually spend time inside my home with my windows open, however sleeping inside still causes me pain in my lung and at times I spit up blood, so it's a serious reaction to something I still can't identify which is very frustrating and I may be forced to sell my home.

The other occasions I have experienced a silent trigger have been outside my home, when I have been away and something was in the air. While I couldn't detect what I was reacting to, I could feel my airway start to restrict, so I listened to and trusted my body giving me the signs and implemented my Plan of Action and left the area. Within a period of time my airway and lung felt a lot better.

Fortunately, this has not happened often and listening to and feeling my body's reaction and implementing my Plan of Action has kept me safe.

Naturally if I am faced with an overwhelmingly big trigger or I react severely to a trigger I cannot smell or taste, then aside from implementing my Plan of Action, I would consider heading to hospital or call an ambulance.

Wind

Where I live, on northerly wind days I generally try to stay inside my home due to the amount of dust and pollutants that get blown around, as it can cause me significant breathing issues. If I do have to go out, I will make sure I wear my masks to help limit the dust.

If the wind is blowing in from the ocean, then I usually drive down to the beach and place my car in a position where I am right next to the beach, getting the ocean air and nothing else. If I go for a walk, I make sure I stay on the ocean side of the road so that car fumes are not blown toward me.

When it's a good wind with no pollutants then I rug up with hat, scarf, gloves and some people look at me as if I'm mad but I will stand or sit breathing in that glorious clean salt air for as long as I can. I call it my free medicine and it makes me feel so very good.

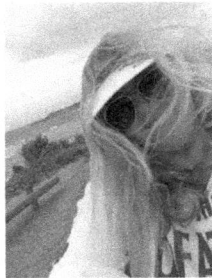

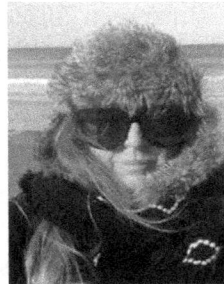

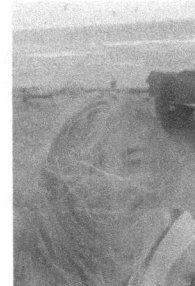

I often speak to people with RADS who have their homes open most days to allow clean air and wind to bellow through their homes. If friends visit my home they know to rug up because I generally have windows and doors open allowing good air flow, so it can be quite cold too.

In my experience and I keep coming back to it *"the movement of clean air"* is a very important factor to my success living with RADS and my overall health and wellbeing.

Winter – Extreme Cold

Although winter used to be my least favorite season, I don't mind the freshness it can create in the air and that's great for my RADS. It's just when it gets really cold it can cause me to have labored breathing and others I have spoken to with RADS have shared having the same experience.

My solution. If I can get away for winter I will and go somewhere not so cold but if I can't, then I just have to suck it up and rug up with a beanie, scarf and jumpers and turn my electric throw rug up a few notches. It can be especially cold sleeping in my van but with enough layers on it's usually just my nose that feels like it has a bit of ice on it. Having warm drinks like lemon and honey can be helpful and soothing on my throat and warm me up!

CHANGING YOUR ENVIRONMENT

If I am planning to go away, I now do research and check if it's fire season, harvest time for farmers, burning-off and what temperatures to expect.

I have spoken to others with RADS who have made the big decision to pack up and move to a new location and environment more beneficial to living with their RADS.

Some have purchased motorhomes or caravans to live in fulltime or part-time and others travel on holidays to seek out the best places to live or stay that are as trigger free as possible. Some people also travel to just get some short-term relief away from polluted environments. Trying to find a place that is just right can be a challenge but please know you are not the only one out there doing it.

Even if you do move and you feel comfortable in your decision, be prepared and expect you may have some challenges. An enormous help to me was renting in the area first and learning where and when I had the best breathing experience.

Living on the Surf Coast had additional challenges of many tourists visiting over summer wearing sunscreen, insect repellent, more vehicle omissions and farmers or council burning off. So, I use all these times as reasons to get away and visit family and friends.

The upsides to living here greatly outweigh the downsides as it is a fantastic place to live. Best of all, when the wind is blowing from the right direction, I have the most amazing salt air cascading off the ocean to breathe in heal and enjoy and its now only minutes away!

I sure hope you find a place to visit, live or stay that has wonderful clean air to breathe and you have many good air days!

IN CLOSING

I must admit it's a little strange finally seeing all my notes from over the years living with RADS finally in a book and crunched down to just a hundred or so pages. It's taken me some time to put together due to having RADS and all the unpredictable anomalies that happen along the way, so thanks for your patience. I am sure there will be additions and updates over the coming years and I look forward to creating Volume 2.

I hope after reading my book it has stirred up determination, enthusiasm and interest in new information that assists you to reduce or eliminate various triggers.

I also hope you are motivated to speak with your medical professional to create a management plan best suited to your specific needs and living with RADS.

If my book has inspired you to start investing time and do the work for positive new beginnings to build a better quality of life living with RADS, then I'm thrilled!

Remember you now have a Super Power in having RADS, so why not make it work for you!

I look forward to a future cure for RADS and wish you all good air days.

Sincerely,

Taryn Bock
radsinternational@gmail.com
www.radsinternational.com
www.breathingissues.weebly.com

PS. It would be wonderful to hear from those who have read my book and would like to provide a review, share feedback or comments for my website. Thanks very much. My email is radsinternational@gmail.com

Books and Programs I Have Found Interesting and Helpful:-

Quantum Healing Hypnosis Academy - QHHT ® - Dolores Cannon

Idiots Guide to Self-Hypnosis – Dr Synthia Andrews, ND

Creative Visualization and Self-Hypnosis – Tim Reid

The Path of Emotions – Dr Synthia Andrews, ND

Freeing the Captives – Louise Ireland-Frey, M.D.

Thank you and Acknowledgements

I would like to say a big thank you to Dr Malin for taking the time to read my book and write such a wonderful Foreword and being a great support to me since my diagnosis. I would also like to thank Dr Badir for his kind words in his review and for his ongoing support.

A heartfelt thankyou to Bev Turner for proof reading and assisting me with editing. Her time and knowledge from her State Registered nursing career and her experience living with multiple chemical sensitivity challenges has been extremely valuable.

Thanks to my mum and to my son for their love and support while I was learning how to live with this condition and for their continued encouragement in any endeavor I undertake.

Many thanks to my brother Phil who has been an especially good listener over the years providing helpful feedback, moral support and great help editing!

Also, thanks to my cousin Lisa in Victoria for being a great sounding board over the years and offering her hospitality and driveway on many occasions as a safe place for me to park my van and sleep.

Thanks to my cousin Lisa in SA who has been there for me via phone at some of my most struggling times.

Thanks to my Uncle and Aunty and all my cousins in WA for their humour, warmth, love, hospitality and looking after me in WA.

Thank you to my lifelong friend Wendy (Peewee) for her unwavering support in helping to run the online groups and her friendship.

Thanks to Melanie and Steven for their guidance and encouragement in publishing my book.

I am also grateful to those family and friends who worked with me in accepting my new rules to maintain friendships, communication and those who went out of their way to accommodate my RADS.

You all know who you are. Xx

About the Author

Taryn lives at the Surf Coast in Victoria, Australia and throughout her working career she held positions that utilized her problem-solving skills and successfully analyzed, designed and implemented various systems in a diverse range of companies. She attended Port Adelaide College of TAFE and became a qualified Trainer to train and guide staff in developing programs to suit a company's needs. As an avid inventor she also created and co-built an occupational health and safety software program called Smidgit ®.

In her private time, she completed two Hypnosis courses and became a Practitioner of Hypnosis focusing on healing. She holds a Diploma in counselling and facilitated and ran grief counselling sessions. She has written a screen play, co-authored a children's feature film and enjoys song writing and production. She is a keen photographer shooting surf photography and landscapes as well as her new puppy!

After being injured and left with RADS, Taryn was isolated and alone and had not met anyone else with RADS. She drew on her work experience and skill set to create successful strategies, tools and solutions to reduce triggers and manage her breathing issues. Her other life passions and interests were paramount in helping to create methods and solutions for her emotional wellbeing and to support her mental health.

Taryn built two websites to share information about her new journey living with RADS, sharing what helped her and what she had learnt from medical professionals.

www.radsinternational.com   and   www.breathingissues.weebly.com

Taryn has supported and mentored others newly diagnosed with RADS since 2015 and does all she can, when she is well, to spread awareness about RADS, as this is something she is extremely passionate about.

www.ingramcontent.com/pod-product-compliance
Lightning Source LLC
Chambersburg PA
CBHW080617270326
41928CB00016B/3096